THE
ANSWERS
ARE
WITHIN

Published in Australia by
Inspire for Life Publishing
coach@inspireforlife.com.au

First published in Australia 2024
Copyright © Anne Poole 2024

National Library of Australia Cataloguing in Publication entry

 A catalogue record for this
book is available from the
National Library of Australia

ISBN 978-1-7635562-0-1 (paperback)
ISBN 978-1-7635562-1-8 (hardback)
ISBN 978-1-7635562-3-2 (epub)

Feather photo by Pam Day UK
Author photo by Karen Cougan
Edited by Karen Crombie at Exact Editing
Layout and design by Sophie White Design

Printed by Ingram Spark

All care has been taken in the preparation of the information
herein, but no responsibility can be accepted by the publisher or
author for any damages resulting from the misinterpretation of
this work. All contact details given in this book were current at the
time of publication, but are subject to change.

The advice given in this book is based on the experience of the
individuals. Professionals should be consulted for individual
problems. The author and publisher shall not be responsible for
any person with regard to any loss or damage caused directly or
indirectly by the information in this book.

The
ANSWERS
Are Within

A Life-Changing, Practical Guide to
Trusting Your Intuition, and Finding Peace
and Joy in Challenging Times

ANNE POOLE

To my precious granddaughters

Lucie Rose Nicole Poole
&
Ava Joyce Poole

Who give me pure joy and much happiness.

To my beautiful goddaughters

Alice Kristina Moore
&
Annette Marie Wood

Gifted and amazing women whom I love dearly.

To my gorgeous Finnish exchange daughter

Sanna Elina Taipale

Talented and loving, lighting up my life.

ABOUT THE AUTHOR

Anne is a lifelong learner. Having endured a "hard" life, she continues to undertake courses to help her academically, socially, spiritually, as well as emotionally.

Anne had a calling to write this book when she faced retrenchment as her manager position was made redundant. It was a perfect segue to reflect on her life before the next direction unfolded. She wanted to inspire and motivate others to know that there is a way forward. She found the answers within. Anne took time to do the inner work and believed in herself. Yes, she had the answers for attaining peace and joy. Calmness within prevailed.

Anne's struggles may not be like yours, yet the emotions will be the same.

Anne shares her highs and lows with vulnerability. This book provides clear examples of how to work through the emotional scale. It has everything to do with how you feel when you get out of your head. **Action Aces** at the end of each chapter will provide the key summary actions.

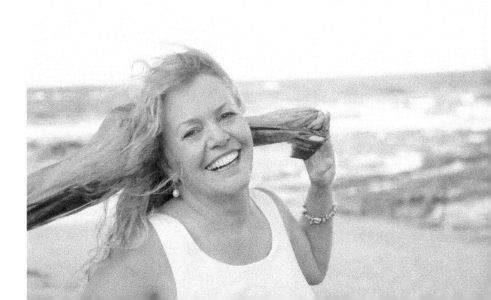

Anne's working life commenced as an Executive Secretary and with further study she gained a Diploma of Business and a Master of Human Resource Management. With a successful career in the Resources Industry, Anne added to her skills a Life Coaching qualification. For the past 15 years she has worked in both fields.

Currently she has programs for Career Advancement and Career Transition. Close to her heart is leadership coaching, as her Girl Guide background set a practical foundation that enabled her to lead high performing corporate teams. Anne's ethos is to position each person for individual and business success.

Anne's love of nature is paramount to her health and happiness. Living on the Cooloola Coast she enjoys walks through the Melaleuca trees and around the beautiful bay and beaches. When she is not writing, she enjoys kicking up her heels on the dance floor!

Stay in touch:

🌐 www.inspireforlife.com.au

f https://www.facebook.com/anne.poole.731

📷 https://www.instagram.com/annabelle813

FOREWORD

Well, I am in tears... your book is so beautiful and your heart shines throughout with love. There is a natural flow as you share with a deep generosity of grace and love for others, opening doors to possibilities, assisting healing. It is in your sharing that the reader recognises aspects and connects gently but powerfully to changes and letting go, empowering health, relationship, joy, and life.

I love the quotes to demonstrate your points at the beginning of each chapter and throughout the book important references, linking up the journey as the reader travels on. Absolutely love your unique style of writing Anne, really, such beautiful choice of words, educated language, and professional presentation. I really enjoyed reading your book, it's so easy to read. Perfect!

You are truly amazing, Anne. I feel a deep appreciation and honour that you have graced me with the gift of reading and feeling everything you have written in your beautiful book. My heart felt the love, I had shivers as I read your Niagara Falls story and the airport farewell with your beloved son; poignant moments of your life generously shared, with no trace of ego, or trying to be anything different, just sharing pure truth to benefit others.

Throughout the highs and lows you share, there is an inner listening and truth that always sustains you, lifting, learning with grace and a thankful heart, to move through difficulties and forward. There is that inner knowing, precious friend, that even the lows cannot take from you. You so clearly demonstrate this, time and time again, and it's so deeply beautiful.

I cried as you recalled the loss of your beloved dad at such a young age, and the pain of your mum's rejection, yet you always feel led by the inner light of Christ leading you on. You draw strength and faith from way beyond this lifetime, a trusted, constant friend in Jesus. I felt your joys and achievements, your work ethic and determination, your appreciation for everything in your life, your love of the natural world, your enthusiasm and hunger to learn. I love your experiences of new things, your visits to new exciting places, fabulous trips and courses throughout the world, your family, friends, work colleagues, and your lovely smile making someone's day.

Nothing is lost on you; the shape of the clouds, a small kindness, a look, a tender moment. The sun shines, beckoning the reader, saying you can be more; the answers are within. Tiny steps start a journey. You inspire, by sharing your amazing journey, never preaching, shoving or pushing, and with this approach, even the most frightened person feels supported, cared for, able, loved, and encouraged to take a step forward...

Your heart knows no bounds, and your wisdom honours your qualities of self-worth and respect, allowing others to feel theirs. In you finding your real You, 'The Answers are Within' is perfect, offering an out-stretched hand of love to others. There is a timeless, exuberant child within you, a wonder and appreciation of all things and people. I am learning so much from your graciousness and gift that we met up again in this lifetime. Across time and space, I know and love you.

Love your dedication to encouraging, supporting, listening, and bonding with groups of people to bring out and enhance their full potential for achieving the highest good. A leader in a million! A true teacher. An answer to a prayer! You provide such an all-inclusive feel to teams and groups that you have managed. Nobody gets overlooked, there's recognition of each person – I see you, hear you, love you.

I admire your empathy... and the courage to share your own experiences of loss and gains. Amongst your many qualities, your ability to listen is one of the richest. For a person to feel truly listened to is rare.

Love the **Action Aces**... beautiful how you have summed things up and given clear points. It feels really positive; yes, I can do that, beautiful!

Pure honesty, a generous heart, self-respect and honour, unconditional love. I feel humbled in your gracious presence. Thank you. I wish you heartfelt and well-deserved success, joy and happiness.

Patricia Dryden

Author, *Soul Poems of Love*

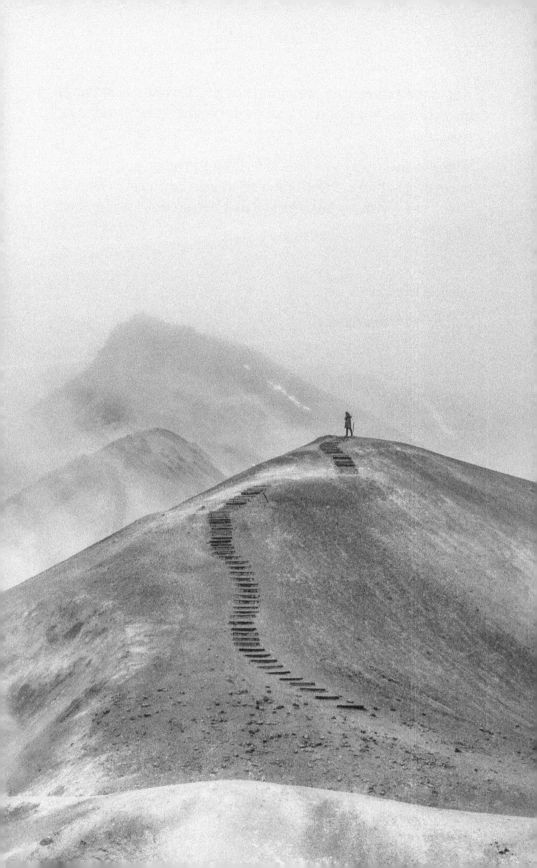

Take The Path Least Travelled

It takes courage and confidence,
It has some risks, but it often brings great rewards:
The challenge of the new,
The thrill of exploration,
Growth from learning
And self-confidence from success.

Patrick Lindsay

I noticed a feather on the ground. I'd gone for a Sunday morning walk. Enraptured, my eyes surveyed the parkland and then focussed on the ground to reveal a myriad of bird feathers scattered amongst the grass. Indeed, was I looking through a magician's mirror?

Suddenly I realised that it was a very long time since I'd appreciated nature.

The colour and variation of feathers was a surprise. The simple elements of nature enthralled me and I collected these feathers as a reminder of this moment – a turning point in my life. I was aware of numerous life changes occurring and that, in the busyness of life, my love of nature and the outdoors had been dormant. Those simple feathers inspired me to live life and to look at all things anew with eyes wide open.

My life at that time was one of turmoil. Full-time employment assisted week to week, yet I didn't have financial security, and I was in a dark place. I was depressed. To assist with my cash flow I applied for a $500 credit card which was declined, as I hadn't lived in my rented unit for more than three months. Previously, I was categorised as an *additional cardholder* and didn't have a credit rating in my own name. Mum had died 12 months earlier, and I was still grieving. I was numb. Emotionally I felt disconnected from life, and all that was occurring impacted my health.

It was during this time of immense change that I was gifted a birthday present of a tattoo. I had always wanted a tattoo, long before it became widely acceptable, and more recently, fashionable. With feathers representing such a symbolic stage of my journey, I decided on American Indian feathers coloured purple and lilac, intertwined with black. When shown the result, I mentioned to the artist that I didn't want red – that was all I could see in the mirror. He kindly explained to me that it was my blood. That colour struck a chord deep within me – I felt alive! Having completed a colour psychology course I was aware that every colour has polarity and red signified fire and blood, energy and danger, strength and power, determination and weakness, passion and indifference, and I was feeling pretty pumped with my tattoo, as well as the feather celebration signalling a shift towards my new direction. Insight for me comes in waves. When I analyse what discernment is, it often presents as a light bulb moment when I recognise and perceive what is occurring. I get an acute realisation or perception of a situation that allows me to make an informed judgement.

After the feather epiphany, I discovered that we choose our parents – a very new concept to me at that time. Abraham Hicks has a great video about this, describing how we make a contract with source energy and we choose a physical experience.[1] This video and explanation is deep and comprehensive. Allow me to summarise how we chose our current physical experience. When I experience a contrasting situation it allows my expansion, a time of growth as things work out for me, as my life has a purpose. There have been times when I questioned things; surely I could not have chosen my parents and these experiences! If I borrow Hicks' analogy of when we walk into a room, there is no dark switch – only the light –

---

1   Abraham Hicks, https://www.youtube.com/watch?v=ulzXaqmSpSs, *Do we choose our parents?*

which we can resist and disallow goodness. Yet I was not always in alignment of good choices and through contrast situations I created my own experience, as I always have a choice. These experiences kept coming back to *me* – my choice to define clearly what I want. It was easy to say that it was another person or external situation that impacted and therefore it was not of my making, and I did that many a time. I *did* have a choice, if I was honest with myself. It has taken me a while to understand that it is just my resistance to what is – and more than ever in these unsettled times, I know resistance does not empower who I am. I have a saying, which you may know, 'Let go and let God.' Some people say, 'Let go and let the universe.' Surrendering to a higher power releases me in that moment. Interestingly, when I accept and feel no resistance, my vibration or frequency, (feeling positive and using my source energy) allows things to work out for me.

I became aware of beliefs that I had never questioned: never understood and blissfully unaware, taken on as my own beliefs. My Oxford Dictionary tells me that a belief is *'a feeling that something exists or its true, especially one without proof; a firmly held opinion; a trust or confidence in; religious faith.'* Belief systems within my mind often have a feeling of absolute certainty and can be empowering beliefs, yet on the flip side I may have a limiting belief because doubt prevails. Empowering beliefs might be that I have absolute clarity on how to make a patchwork quilt and my belief allows me to make the quilt. Limiting beliefs might be that because I don't have enough time, I cannot write a manuscript to publish my book. In both of these scenarios, I had a choice and each decision shaped the outcome based on how I felt. My strong belief was that I could make the quilt, my body and mind aligned, and excitement pulsed my energy as I undertook the various stages to complete the article.

At times, when writing this manuscript, it seemed difficult as my paid work was super busy and my writing often went on the backburner or the words didn't populate the page when I sat at my laptop. Interestingly, my physical state had low energy during these unproductive writing times. I became aware that beliefs shaped a conditioning of my mind as these thoughts were told over and over to me during my formative years, often subconsciously taking hold as I grew older, through my own repetition. I accepted the beliefs my parents told me, as well as what my teachers and youth group leaders had taught. It was the start of a journey to further self-discovery and observing my beliefs. One of my spiritual teachers, Mike Robinson, would say, 'Don't take my word for it – find out for yourself!' Just as this book will give you insights into what is possible, it will also encourage you to believe in yourself – whatever it is you wish to find, the answers are within.

I recognised new awakenings to different concepts and challenged the journey that I had embarked on as an eighteen-year-old girl. The Scout Association of Queensland nominated me as their representative for Miss Youth Week. One of the five panel members enquired about what I wanted to do with my life? My response was to travel and to find myself as an individual. The follow-up question was along the lines of what are you doing towards achieving that? My response was that within one month of judging, I was leaving on a planned six-month overseas trip, commencing with a short attendance at the International Scout Jamboree in Lillehammer, Norway. I was selected as the Miss Youth Week winner and my community work and achievements contributed to this success. At that age I had already read books such as Norman Vincent Peale's *The Power of Positive Thinking*, Louise Hay's *You Can Heal Your Life* and Kahlil Gibran's *The Prophet*, all of which opened my mind to different philosophies. Since then I have remained an avid reader, with an overabundance of books to explore.

As a young woman, this was a time of awakening; this mysterious change was whispering deep within me. At the time, I could not comprehend the magnitude of change ahead of me, yet I knew that I was embarking on an intense soul-searching journey to bring self-healing.

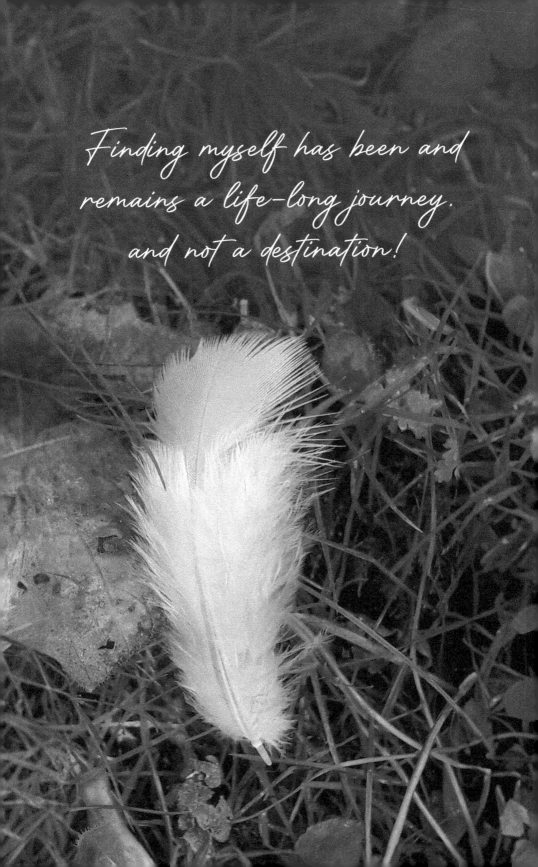

Finding myself has been and
remains a life-long journey.
and not a destination!

CONTENTS

CHAPTER ONE

Introduction and Self-Sustaining Model

*"The story we tell
is the reality we live."*

Lisa Bloom, Story Coach, 16 Sept 2019

When I was only six and a half, my carefree and playful existence abruptly fell apart. Dad went into hospital to deal with a medical condition and unexpectedly died of a heart attack. For my sister and I, there was no funeral. My auntie told us of our dad's death one week after the event. Mum struggled as a sole parent in the 1960s, and it climaxed when she collapsed in the hallway a short time after dad's passing. I was terrified. I kept calling out to her, and there was no response. I envisaged being left alone with only my sister. I used a chair to reach the highest shelf in the kitchen cupboard to find the Smelling salts and carefully used these to bring mum around.

Life had changed and I wondered, why me? I wanted to be daddy's little girl, and questioned if I had done something wrong, for him to leave us? Was there something lacking within me? Was I not worthy to have parents? Mum told us, *'Don't tell people that I'm a widow.'* I didn't understand why. I carried her shame about the situation, and my confusion only grew. The pain of my father's passing stayed with me for a very long time.

I remember that wanting to be loved and to belong were so important that in grade two at school, I sought attention. One day in the playground a lost purse was discovered. It circulated the classrooms, and we were all asked – do you own this purse? I put up my hand to say it was mine, even though it wasn't. The teacher spoke to me about my dishonesty. I felt humiliated, and although the teacher was compassionate towards me because I was grieving the death of my father, I felt shame. It added to my sense of loss and feeling alone.

Has there been a time when you felt unworthy? Even though you did your best, it was not enough? Others did not accept you, and because of that, your stomach was churned up and the situation played out in non- acceptance of yourself? Did you feel that your voice lost its volume or words did not spring forth? Times when self-doubt clouded your focus and hindered you moving forward? Has there been a time when staying put and in denial seemed a better choice than taking the step forward? There are moments in my life when I have felt untalented and not able to meet others' expectations of me. I spiralled into negative thinking and feeling that I couldn't achieve my dreams and goals. I just didn't believe in *me.*

I noticed others achieving career advancement, yet I felt that I wasn't good enough. I was overlooked and not considered. When I felt like this, it impacted all the things that mattered – my work and my relationships.

I did a lot of reading and searching. I found appropriate courses and sought out people to assist me. Step by step, I was gaining a better image of myself and making gradual changes through my thoughts, feelings and actions.

I learned about passive, assertive and aggressive communication styles and how they play out in everyday speech. This information allowed me to improve my communication style and identify the different external interactions.

Communication has changed globally – and continues to evolve. I became part of global communities who moved into the technology era where new technologies, new industries, new educational learning paths and skills overtook those which once provided an income, leaving them obsolete. I felt that I needed to change or at least work out what I could do to exist comfortably in a world where change was constant. Professions which previously guaranteed a ' job for life' were disappearing and being replaced with either automated equipment or being absorbed within other roles. For example, I was a trained bank teller, and Automatic Telling Machines mainly replaced these positions. I was also in the secretarial field. A large number of these positions were reduced through automated processes and those that remained encompassed complex administration at an executive level. These are just a few examples that impacted my life and my sense of self-worth. Advancements in technology mean we have long shifted focus away from work with our hands. Knowledge work – the work of the head – which boomed in the 1980s and '90s meant that cognitive occupations increased at four times the pace of manual labour in Australia.[2]

We are now in the social media phenomenon, which represents a whole new level of instant communication. Even now, I wonder how long our written words will be available for others to see. Potentially social media will have an indefinite timeframe to access my photos, captions and views. Facebook recently notified me that I had attained ten years of participation and produced some memories for me in celebration! How ironic.

I became aware that I live in a fluid society. Today's generation, Gen Z, born 1995 to 2015, appear to feel that life is like their smart phone. When I observe this age group, it is like a fast card game of Snap. Click: transported to another environment via the electronic world; click: instant responses. Friends and I observe

---

2   Kate Neilson, *HRM September 2019*, Issue 58, p14 – Australian Human Resources Institute

younger people at dinner and notice many of the attendees looking at their phone instead of their table mates. Their fingers move quickly, texting to make responses and not miss a single opportunity that has just arisen. Other generations like the Baby Boomers, born 1944 to 1964, may have difficulty communicating because hearing loss is an invisible disability. My main observation is that as people move quickly from one environment to another; they do not necessarily take proper advantage of the face to face communication opportunity.

The busyness of life kept my mind occupied. With so much at my fingertips, I can quickly fill my day with 'information' via social media. I know that if I check my social media, an hour can soon be gone. Social media also provided a disconnect as much as a connection. Measuring myself through the number of 'likes' definitely impacted me on days when I felt unworthy and compared myself to others. Thankfully, changes made to social media limited the visuals so that our value is not automatically measured for all to see. Now, each account owner can quickly check the 'likes' numbers for their page. For some, it is not of interest: for others, it can significantly impact their self-worth.

I have witnessed that in my everyday life things are not usually a click: move forward. I find myself juggling with change constantly, and sometimes I become bogged down. Often decisions are required, and while some can be instant, other times, I need reflection time or time for my inner self to guide me. My intuition or gut feeling or inner compass gives me reliable answers which ultimately reinforce believing in myself. Is it about the world, social media, or is it me; am I truly not good enough? Is it a lie? People can be harsh in their comments and deduce outcomes that are not necessarily entirely correct. At some stages in life, yes, I have believed I am not good enough. I know that I am not alone, and you might be feeling this too. This book will help you to improve that situation now.

It will help you take courageous steps to move forward. You will realise that believing in yourself will give you the confidence to remove the self-doubt and this book will assist you in finding your voice and in knowing you are very worthy. The greatest gift you can give yourself is to invest in *you* – you are the only one who can make these changes, with support from mentors, coaches and people who want the best for you.

Friends have said that my life has been hard: one where I have dug deep to work through the emotions and move through the feelings that fear represents. Fear presents in many guises – like frustration and anger. I have found acceptance in even the most difficult of my situations. I have a strong determination to meet my own goals, and profound courage to face all that my life journey brings and embrace the lessons it has taught me.

Each of us has a life journey, and people and events are part of the process to help us on the way. Sometimes when life seems incredibly harsh, there often is a silver lining – although we may not believe or see it at the time. Reflection is excellent to evaluate the bigger picture – how things unfolded through the choices I made. I have learned to choose the options carefully in every moment.

I now live a happy and fulfilled life. I believe in me. This book will provide tools and real life examples to illustrate transformational change. Now is the perfect time to find the answers within. You can read this book from start to finish, or find the chapter which speaks to you and plunge into the stories and tools. Now is the perfect time to believe in you and find the answers within. Do not just select click for the next instalment: take time to reflect and get clear on your goals and start believing in your inner self.

Each chapter has *Action Aces* to summarise the salient points and a call to take action. Gain traction on what you want to improve in your life; it is essential to be **consistent** in the application of the changes you make. While it is great to learn about new tools and read another's story, it is vital for your success that you commit to action every day. Write down one thing each day you wish to achieve and do it! Then add another item that you want to accomplish and build on it. By focussing on one action daily, you will remove feelings of being overwhelmed. Small and regular activity outweighs a random grand gesture every time. Consistency will bring success. Be successful!

You may find slight repetition in different chapters. If you did a deep dive on only one chapter, it is not necessary to have read previous chapters. If you are reading it sequentially, it will reinforce the importance.

The book is a platform to allow you to feel good, have fun and release joy. Remember, acceptance is the ability to have a clear view of how things are and being present. Find your quiet determination that 'I am not my circumstance; what's happening around me does not define me.' Have a clear vision for reaching a better place – to do, to be, to live, to experience beautiful things.

I know that the book will help you to find **The Answers Are Within**. My greatest wish is that whatever resonates within you will be your calling – take up the challenge and deliver joy to yourself. This book is for you – choose you!

With love.

Anne x

CHAPTER TWO

Feeling Unhealthy – Gaining Vitality

*"A healthy outside
starts from the inside."*

Robert Urich

Well over twenty-five years ago, I embarked on a ritual of picking up my two sons from childcare and then popping into the bakery to collect some afternoon tea. I'd eagerly wait to see the boys and also have a cream bun – the ones with fresh cream. Wow, what a treat each weekday, and after a while, I found that one didn't fill me – I wanted two cream buns. Soon, two became three cream buns. This went on for a very long time until we moved location and suddenly there were no bakery shops that supplied fresh cream buns. I was devastated. My body changed during that time – I had developed love handles on my hips – the cream found a home and my weight ballooned. I clearly remember trying on a lovely outfit, and the sales assistant advised that I must have my underwear caught up as there was this bulge... no, it wasn't underwear bunched up, it was a cream love handle. Oh, dear. What an ah-hah moment. The cream buns were providing comfort to me, and while they did the trick for an afternoon delight, they masked what was going on inside me. I was unhappy.

Have you ever used food or an alcoholic beverage to fulfil you?

Similarly, purchasing a new pair of shoes, a handbag or a new outfit makes you feel good for a short while, yet it does not sustain you.

If you can relate to these purchase profiles, you will immediately understand that it only temporarily fills the void. Martin Seligman explains that despite the delights that these sensations bring, we often require more significant doses to deliver the same state and over time these feelings diminish.[3] Positive Psychology Today explains it as hedonistic happiness and in its essence, is a brief experience of joy and pleasure which quickly fades away.[4] For example, when you eat a delicious chocolate cake, you get the short-lived feeling of comfort spreading through your body – that's fleeting happiness.

I became aware through reading and reflection that my emotional turmoil manifested itself through a physical condition. And I became aware of the emotions I was unable or unwilling to express outwardly, which may have contributed to my poor health. It felt as though my organs were carrying this considerable weight, physically and emotionally, which was impacting every aspect of my life.

At the time, I didn't have the skills to realise why I was comfort eating. This habitual sweet eating was an early warning sign that something was not flowing in my life. When I got honest with myself, quite some years later, and once that realisation occurred, I knew I had to make a change with my life.

Emotionally it was a turbulent period. I shed a lot of tears. I felt confused. I felt my life was like a washing machine – washed inside out, round and about, and wrung out to dry. I was subjected to lots of comments from family and friends, both supportive and non-supportive. Yet, it was a mixture of my beliefs, my fear, plus their

---

3   Martin Seligman, 2002, *Authentic Happiness*, Ch 7 p103–104
4   https://www.psychologytoday.com/au/blog/mindfulness-wellbeing/201603/why-is-happiness-fleeting

projected fears and conditioning, which let me take a new look at life. Inspiration whispered to me during one particular walk in nature and from this insight I took action and attended a week intensive on process-orientated psychology, as well as connecting with a regular meeting group of like-minded people. The timing was perfect.

I recall an event when certain critical words about not being a good mother felt like I had been punched in the stomach. In essence, being a mother was the greatest blessing and I have always loved my sons unconditionally. In my distressed emotional state, I took on these words of anger. I reached an incredibly low point after that conversation and en route back to my unit, I felt drawn to drive my car into the Brisbane River. I could drown my sorrows and emotions and leave the pain behind me, yet my two sons were uppermost in my thoughts. Instead, I continued driving to my rented unit. On arriving home, I engaged in a very long, cold shower, followed by warm water and visualised filling myself with white light. The tears dripped their blood amongst the cold water. My head throbbed; my eyes were slits peeking through painfully swollen eyelids. I did feel slightly better for releasing these emotions.

If you ever feel someone might be suicidal, talk to them. Just being there and listening is the most important conversation. One way to bring this up is along the lines of:

'I've noticed that you haven't been yourself lately, is everything okay with you? I'm concerned about you. I'm wondering if we can talk about what's troubling you? You've seemed real... down... sad... angry... unhappy... lately. I'm worried that you might be thinking of hurting yourself or suicide. Can we talk about this?'[5]

---

5   Mindstar.com.au, 2019, *Suicide-Prevention*

Genuine interest to get them talking will assist greatly – do not take no for an answer. Many organisations exist around the world where free counselling is available. Share local information with your friend. Seeking help is paramount. Remember you do not need to be ready with answers or perfect solutions; simply be willing to listen and encourage them to access professional support.

Before this event, my naturopath Miriam, suggested supplements as well as the concept to remove negativity through cold showers. Scientific evidence has proven the benefits of cold showers.[6] Remember a time when you enjoyed a swim in the ocean, and as you emerged from the water, you felt terrific. That very same feeling occurs with cold showers. Cold showers improve circulation and strengthen the immune system.[7] Ideally taking a cold shower first thing in the morning is a great way to invigorate yourself for the day ahead. It is also beneficial to take a cold shower (followed by warm water) after being out and about with lots of people around. Furthermore, just before bed take a cold shower, as it clears the mind as well as aiding rest and deep sleep. When introducing any change to your lifestyle, it takes approximately 28 days to become a habit. If you follow through this suggestion, you will notice that there is a difference – it's in the feeling.

If you live near the sea or perhaps have access to the ocean, that is even better. Saltwater is amazing, providing so many health benefits it is sometimes referred to as Vitamin Sea.[8] The article speaks of the overall psychological health benefits, from being in the seawater and the skin absorbing the magnesium and other minerals, to improving the respiratory system. If the sea is not an option, try standing under cold water for a minimum of 10 seconds, ensuring water goes across the nape of the neck and also across the forehead (third eye). Follow by warm water and visualising golden or white light to expand the warmth. Repeat daily to feel the

6   Mike Robinson, 2010, *The True Dynamics of Life*, p205-207
7   https://www.wimhofmethod.com/benefits-of-cold-showers
8   https://www.nib.com.au/the-checkup/health-benefits-of-sea-water

full health benefits. It costs nothing – just your time and mindset change to action this fantastic remedy. For some people, there may be an adverse reaction in that the cold water causes a sharp intake of breath which in turn may potentially accelerate the heart rate and increase blood pressure. Check with a naturopath or doctor if uncertain.

When we interact with others, we are affected by all that is around us. Their thoughts, emotions and feelings come into our energy field. Clearing our cells can provide the change that is required. We have an etheric field surrounding our whole body, which transmits transverse waves of energy. It can be called our aura which extends approximately one to two metres around us. Each cell in our body contains water which can absorb and retain memory. Water is yin and cold is yin. Therefore, from a Chinese yin and yang point of view, the double yin is quite powerful. If you are not familiar with yin and yang, my simple version is that it comes from ancient Chinese philosophy and embodies the concept of dualism and how seemingly opposite forces may be complementary. Yin is feminine, and Yang is masculine, and these opposites interrelate to one another.

After my relationship ended, I was not coping well. I exhibited many signs of depression and as a result visited my local doctor, known in Australia as a General Practitioner (GP). I was sad, my sleep patterns were erratic, significant weight loss occurred and my thoughts of being worthless surfaced from time to time. For a short phase, anti-depressant medication assisted with my functioning and coping with day-to-day activities. Each of us may face depression in our lifetime or be aware of someone showing the signs. I have found it worthwhile seeking help from professionals. Sometimes it is because of a sudden event or situation which hugely impacts us for a relatively short time, yet it feels longer. And for some, it is a longer-term state.

Another tool that helped my anxious state was focussed breathing

– it helps still the mind. To gain the most out of breathing exercises, find a quiet place to sit up straight – aligned posture assists deep breathing, relax with your hands on your lap with palms facing upwards. To begin, it is important to slowly exhale before taking a very deep breath through your nose through to your solar plexus area (around your navel) and fill your abdomen while counting to four. Hold the breath and count to four. Slowly breathe out your mouth, again counting to four. This is known as the Box Method and you will feel more centred within yourself and you will find that calmness fills you if you repeat this process four times.[9] It is important to keep concentration on the breath: if the mind strays, bring it back to your breathing. There are many variations on this, yet a proven and simple technique to provide immediate calmness is the '3, 2, 5 breathe' pattern. After an initial exhale, breathe in for the count of three, hold for two and exhale for five, repeat.

Looking after my health became paramount and I attended courses about aromatherapy to understand natural herbs and applications. Getting back to simple remedies was high on my list to improve my wellbeing. Lavender oil was utilised to calm and soothe me as well as promote better sleep. Many other oils assisted and there are books explicitly dedicated to the use of natural oils which I recommend exploring.

My habits changed. I commenced the day with a cup of hot water with the juice of half a freshly squeezed lemon. This combination kick-starts the liver and assists the body's digestive system, promoting a natural antiseptic and helps flush out impurities in the body. More recently I've introduced celery juice first thing on an empty stomach and then thirty minutes or so later I will have my lemon drink. Celery juice gets into the cells in the body and keeps going deeper. I have noticed with the celery juice that I have better thought clarity and recall of information, plus overall good health.

---

9   https://www.healthline.com/health/box-breathing

I also became more aware of drinking water. Most of us are blessed with easy access to water and often in our busyness, we overlook hydrating our body. Whatever your views on tap water or quality filtered water, consume water to benefit your internal organs. We often substitute coffee and tea for our social drinks with friends, yet that doesn't count as drinking water. Instead, try having a cup of hot water when meeting with others... cafes are happy to oblige when I'm on a detox. It is amazingly good. I might add that I am a bit of a stickler for putting fresh water into the kettle. Many years ago, I listened to a reputable science program with Dr Karl Kruszelnicki, AM, who spoke about keeping the oxygen in the water and not to boil it over and over, as this depletes the oxygen and then there is no oxygen to 'extract' the delicate tea or coffee flavours. Hence, I only use fresh water and just enough for the required number of cups. Having a cup of hot water alone is perfect during the autumn and winter seasons.

When drinking water, it is better for your body to consume it at room temperature. Room temperature varies where you may live, yet it is accepted that a range from twenty to twenty-two degrees Celsius or sixty-eight to seventy-two degrees Fahrenheit is considered room temperature. Cold water can be refreshing on a very hot day, yet it may cause the heart rate to decrease, whereas room temperature water maintains hydration.

Consider consuming two litres of water a day to improve your health through drinking water or through some of the many foods which have a large component of water – such as watermelon. There are many schools of thought on how much water to drink. When passing urine, check the colour and if it is clear, you are drinking enough water. A darker urine colour usually signifies that your water consumption is not enough. Our kidneys can eliminate quite a bit over twenty-four hours. Do your research and work out what is ideal for your height and size and your activity levels. Whatever way you go, please start the twenty-eight day change now to begin your new habit and drink one to two litres per day. The equivalent is about four to eight glasses of water per day. If you are already doing this – well done!

Spending time tending my garden assisted my health – fresh air, sunshine, and hands in the soil. Time in the sunshine is paramount to good health. Often, to protect ourselves when spending long periods in the sun, we are advised to apply UV (Ultraviolet rays) protection –great advice for many Australians who work and play outdoors. When I was working long hours – often leaving home at six am and returning close to six pm – I didn't get outside to feel the sunshine at all. My Vitamin D levels plummeted. My doctor suggested I get out into the sun and take some supplements. I also know that sun exposure on the nostrils is like applying nature's antiseptic as it cleanses and heals. I have found that five to ten minutes of sunshine each day can makes a world of difference to my health. Scientifically it has been said that the UV rays of the sun help your body make this nutrient, assisting your immune system. Scientists debate the amount of sunshine required, because of many variables. Become aware of what is suitable for where you live and whether your skin type requires more or less exposure.[10] If you are fortunate enough to have a yard and garden, then sunshine should be part of your week in the outdoors.

Getting my hands in the soil was also a wonderful activity to connect with nature and feel the absolute joy of looking after a seedling or plant. Sometimes overwhelming anxiety crept in before I commenced gardening and internally, I would raise the question: where do I start? I have learned that doing a little each week helps considerably. While watering the plants, I would pull out a weed that became obvious. As I was doing my gardening chores, I observed that a vine – a weed – was tangled through many branches of my beautiful native trees. As I was intently removing the vine from the tree, I thought of the analogy to my tangled life. Times when I felt

---

10 https://www.ncbi.nlm.nih.gov/pmc/articles/PMC5129901/

bound by public opinion; times when I felt pressured and did not take a stance, times when I was paralysed by fear, and times when I did not honour myself. Subsequently it felt like the vine voyaging all over my vulnerability. As I kept removing the vine, each plant specimen required a similar approach. Cutting the vine at strategic points, and then pulling through the many ends to remove its stranglehold. In my life, I have found this symbolic of cutting the cord technique – a process to remove a person from my life because I have changed energetically. Each energetic interaction I have with someone enables cords to form. These cords or ties may become quite harmful, even choking, and I can feel drained after being in that person's company.

One technique that has worked for me is to imagine standing in the middle of a blue disk with a large radius. Close your eyes and visualise cutting or severing the cord from you and gently tossing the cord away from the disk. If you are familiar with the chakras – visualise pulling or cutting away any cords, commencing with the crown chakra, third eye, throat, heart, solar plexus, sacral, and base. Then move into the liver, spleen, heart, kidneys, base of spine and back of the spine and around the neck. With each area, cut away or pull through any cords. Once visualised and you feel all the cords are gone, carefully check that none remain on the blue disk. Then envision lighting a flame around the disk circle and let it grow higher until it is above your head. When you feel cleansed, slowly become aware of your toes, and wriggle your fingers and open your eyes. Repeat this symbolic cutting for three consecutive days to break the flow of energy between the person and you, or until you feel it has dissipated. This process is about letting go of the old—those people who do not support nor serve you any longer. The negativity is removed from your life. Please be mindful that this energetic exercise will impact the person you are removing.

When transformation occurs gradually, it impacts all aspects of the person – physical, mental, emotional and spiritual. I was aware that during the divorce, my stress levels were high. I attended a detoxification program where I learned about the alkaline acid eighty/ twenty food theory rule, whereby alkaline and acidic food forms an ash residue after metabolism.[11] Hippocrates healed his patients in ancient times utilising dietary recommendations based on foods that leave an ash residue. Depending on the mineral composition of the food and how each individual digests them, our ups and downs in life impact the ash residue after metabolism. Stress and negative emotions, plus poor food choices, can produce acidic residues. To obtain alkalizing results, research and implement the best food combinations. Moderate quantities of food chewed well, along with relaxation, moderate exercise, as well as meditation or prayer, being centred and acts of kindness all combine to achieve alkaline results. Citrus tastes acidic, yet some varieties leave an alkaline residue. Some fruits and vegetables which are highly alkaline forming are lemons, watermelon, cantaloupe, mango, papaya, parsley, asparagus, carrots and celery. Gradual changes to my diet assisted my overall good health and minimised any cleansing or healing crisis. Much is written about 'super foods' to support good health and I encourage you to be open to researching good local food for the climate in which you live and foods that replenish the levels of your active or non-active life.

I gifted myself detox juicing retreats and further honoured this time with nurturing walks and swims in the ocean. It was a time to contemplate, to share with others, to experience new juice recipes, to visualise the inner change that such vitamins and minerals would bring through the juicing process. I listened to meditations. Because my physical being was changing, the dynamics of my emotions felt like musical scales punctuated with a crescendo. The detox provided many food changes which assisted and cleared the toxins from my physical body. During the process, I cried buckets, releasing the emotional toxins. I did the inner work – a term I use

11 Food Theory Chart adapted *"Alkalize or Die"* by Dr T Baroody, Holographic Health, USA

for just allowing time to make observations, to really feel and accept my emotional state and then progress my healing. Gradually I peeled away and discarded a plethora of old beliefs; giving way to knowing the real Anne.

Juicing has become part of my lifestyle. I regularly have the discipline to action either fourteen, twenty-one, or twenty-eight day juice cleanses. No alcohol or coffee is permitted during this detox period. My doctor commented that my blood results are excellent and to 'Keep doing what you are doing because it is working!' I have found that undertaking a detox twice yearly for fourteen days each time has improved my health and wellbeing.

Notably, when I first commenced a detox program, my emotional state see-sawed. I was shown a way to release emotions through Mike Robinson's 11 x 22s.[12] At the time, with my feelings frayed, I felt life was giving me lemons at each turn. Applying a tool to assist this inner work was to focus on affirmative 'I' sentences and then release whatever the mind conjures onto paper for each of these twenty-two sentences in the daily session. I used the positive sentence for wellbeing: 'I am well and healthy…' This process occurred for eleven days. The **'Action Aces'** section will provide more details on how to do this exercise.

11 x 22s are compelling numbers, which, when used as a healing tool, bring dramatic change. The process of using numbers with repeated affirmative sentences did break down some of my belief patterns. Further changes occurred within my emotional state as well as my physical body. On an energetic level, the positive words entered into the mind and body, pushing out the distorted energy through the words which followed. An internal shift occurred as the distortion was dispersed through my aura, leaving it clear. I would do many of these 11 x 22s in the following fifteen years, expressing feelings onto paper and then destroying: a powerful release method.

---

12 Mike Robinson, 2002 *The True Dynamics of Relationships*, p311–316

It is important not to read again what you have written. Remove the paper with the written words from your dwelling – either through burning or soaking in water and emptying into the rubbish bin externally. You can type this, yet it is more powerful when you handwrite. It is essential not to miss a day; if you do, start again. These simple exercises were powerful and greatly assisted on my journey to improving my overall health.

Undertaking a detox program affects every cell in your body. You may not have given it a great deal of thought, and you may not feel drawn to the self-care required in this personal program. It is a commitment and enforced discipline to achieve a high level of wellbeing.

Eating fresh fruit and vegetables, adding fish and some meat, a personal choice, made a big difference to my overall wellbeing. Whenever practical, I sourced organic vegetables or pesticide free, as it is undoubtedly better for your health. Local markets supply fresh, good quality produce at affordable prices. I kept my budget in focus by planning my weekly meals and sought seasonal fruit and vegetables to get variety in my recipes. While I have lots of cookbooks – these are beneficial – these days I can easily find good recipes online. Find out about alkaline vegetables and fruit and have eighty percent of your meals with these ingredients. Consider changes to your diet as it can make a subtle or big health difference, depending on your current status. I am not an expert in nutrition, but I am an avid cook who enjoys preparing tasty, easy meals that allow my body and mind to function to capacity.

I experienced bad breath before starting on my first detox. This can be for several reasons and not just having garlic in the previous meal! For me, it was more about my gut health or lack of good gut health. It's important to understand that the microbiome in the gut affects our brain as well as every aspect of our health.[13] Probiotics

---

13 https://www.healthline.com/nutrition/gut-microbiome-and-health

prescribed by a naturopath or similarly qualified nutritionist assist with maintaining good gut health. I also undertook enemas during the detox program as this supported the removal of waste from the large intestine. For over ten years I have found colon hydrotherapy an excellent way to keep my colon clear. Some benefits include an improved digestive function, increased general hydration, an increase to energy levels, weight loss; improved sleeping patterns and refined concentration and clarity.

It's very interesting how our internal health can impact the skin – our external appearance. For example, a friend went on a carrot detox for several weeks and her skin colour had an orange tinge. This is extreme yet definitely possible. What we ingest can sometimes show up through our skin. I know if I over-indulge in chocolate, I might get a pimple on my face. Sometimes though, our skin condition is impacted through our genes. As the years go by, I have realised that taking care of my skin has become a priority. To keep my skin in its best condition, I ensure that I cleanse and moisturise, both morning and night. Previously, I had struggled with this regime. Now with fabulous devices and plant-based products, I love the freshness of my skin and it only takes a few minutes a day to maintain. This is definitely a daily habit.

I have always maintained good oral health. Each of us can do a quick brush of our teeth and maybe a floss, yet regular new toothbrushes make a big difference. Do you also brush your tongue? I have found it worthwhile. I seek professional dental attention at least yearly and often every six months. Good dentists are more pro-active in assisting our oral hygiene and defer immediate action unless there is a direct impact on our health. If funds are tight and dental check-ups become pushed out, definitely utilise dental floss. It works wonders for regular maintenance of your gums and removal of unwanted food lodged between teeth.

When I think of oral health, I automatically think of my talented dentist and his professional care. He appreciates my smile – it is such an easy thing to share with people. As I travelled the world, I may not have known the language, yet a smile from me sparks a mutual nodding of acknowledgment. A smile is free. It does exercise the muscles, whereas a frown takes a lot more muscles to produce. A smile can break down barriers and internally, it makes us feel good! Try it out yourself to find out.

Throughout the years, I have undertaken an ancient method of cleansing the mouth called Oil Pulling. You may or may not be familiar with this terminology. Dr Karach provides a good explanation:

"Oil pulling is very simple, completely harmless, and inexpensive, unlike most medical treatment. The cost is the price of a daily spoonful of vegetable oil —cheaper than even a vitamin tablet. Yet, it is one of the most powerful forms of therapy."[14]

Alternatively, you can use sesame oil, and from my experience, a good quality cold-pressed organic coconut oil works well. Healthy Atom, who organised many of my detox programs explains the theory of this science:

"Oil is non-polar and attracts non-polar molecules. The arrangement or geometry of the atoms in some molecules is such that one end of the molecule has a positive electrical charge and the other has a negative charge. If this is the case, the molecule is called a polar molecule, meaning that it has electrical poles. Otherwise, it is called a non-polar molecule. Whether molecules are polar or non-polar determines if they will mix to form a solution.

Saliva, which is secreted into the mouth when the oil is repeatedly swished and pulled is mainly composed of water, electrolytes, digestive enzymes, antibacterial and antifungal/ antiviral agents. These are

---

14 http://www.oilpulling.com/

predominantly polar and therefore attract polar molecules. It is this heterogeneous mixture that works together to rid the mouth and body of unwanted toxins and chemicals."[15]

The **Action Aces** section at the end of this chapter provides the process. I found it very worthwhile as well as an economical, practical, and easy way to cleanse toxins from my mouth.

Regular exercise also aids good overall health. I commenced with walking for about 30 mins a day and then extended the time and pace. It is recommended, for most of us, that we undertake 10,000 steps a day. I recall my time in the Girl Guides, when we regularly learned and participated in *'Scout's Pace'*. This involved walking from one telegraph pole (now known as an electricity pole) to the next and then running to the next pole and then walking to the next pole, and so on. At the start, we received a message we were required to convey on return. Our brain was engaged. There was a lot of laughter with the returned messages as they often became somewhat scrambled! Nowadays not as many electricity poles are visible as the gas and electricity services are often underground, so perhaps you could use another landmark which will signify a change of pace. What this example conveyed is the methodology of walk... run... walk... run, which builds our stamina as well as assists with our breathing, especially if starting anew with an exercise program. If you are competitive, you can monitor the distance versus time ratios. Give it a try and experience it for yourself. Having a mindset to believe you can do the walk... run... skip... jog... bicycle ride, makes a huge difference. Our state of mind, and how people around us influence that, will impact the effectiveness of the activity.

Whatever is occurring for you, it is always essential that you follow your heart or intuition as then you are freeing yourself, and the joy will flow. Another exercise I love is Latin dance. Regular

---

15 https://www.healthyatom.com/index.php?route=common/home

attendance at classes improved my life socially as well as mentally and physically. Published longitudinal studies in 2003, with a cohort of 469 subjects aged over 75 years, found that dancing can reduce the onset of dementia.[16] It measured each participant's mental alertness as a means of monitoring rates of dementia, including Alzheimer's Disease. The research program covered a range of cognitive and physical activities. Activities included playing cards, walking, dancing, tennis, swimming, golf, musical instruments, reading, and crossword puzzles. Surprisingly, dance was one activity that was good for the mind, significantly reducing dementia risk. Dance also helps alleviate symptoms of Parkinson's disease. The study further cited that *'the Argentine Tango can improve an individual's spatial awareness and memory because of the postures and simple paths learned during the dance classes.'*[17] Dancers store these sequences in a neural pathway. It is remembered and used again, and, significantly, it is equally important for individuals to improvise and respond spontaneously to the music. Often when a leader (usually a male) directs the follower (often a female), it is the follower who takes the cues and moves spontaneously. The leader can change the sequence in many of the dance routines to suit the music, and this allows the brain to open many neural pathways. The article further quotes research by Neurologist Dr Robert Katzman. He says that dances like foxtrot, waltz and swing that require the rapid- fire and constant split-second decision making are vital in maintaining intelligence. It forces your brain to rewire the neural pathways, which delivers greater cognitive reserve regularly. There are so many dances to enjoy! Each has different learning steps with routines and even with two left feet, there is line dancing, which is rote learned and enjoyable.

Select an activity that brings you joy. It's a great idea to attend different events to find which one lights you up internally.

---

16 New England Journal of Medicine
17 http:// blogs.biomedcentra l.com/bmcseriesblog/2016/04/04/keep-dancing-turns-good-brain/

The process of gaining vitality is like a 360-degree look at our everyday habits. All that activity requires sleep and rest. Sleep is such a vital part of attaining and maintaining good inner health. Have you ever noticed when you are sleep deprived, that your otherwise good vibe has disappeared? I found with lack of sleep my usual happy-go-lucky vibe has a shorter wick. My experience when I have not had a good night's sleep is that comments which I previously would have laughed along with or tolerated now bring emotions of annoyance and irritability. A lot of the time, if we have a substantial diet, engage in exercise, and enjoy social activities, sleep occurs soon after our head hits the pillow. If you'd like to read further, this article is very comprehensive. https://www.helpguide. org/harvard/biology-of-sleep-circadian-rhythms-sleep-stages.htm

When we go to sleep, there are wavelengths which occur and through my awareness, I share:

Beta	uuuuuuuu active consensus close together
Alpha	u u u u
Theta	u u} Between Theta and Delta is REM (rapid eye movement)
Delta	u u u u u u u u} = sleep

When I face significant decisions or changes in my life, I wake at early hours in the morning. Often, the concern, issue or problem is being played over and over again in my head. I remember times when I had a considerable workload, I was waking up and recalling all the little things to include the next day at work. For example, I must remember to do that correspondence or make that phone call. Is that true for you?

There are many schools of thought about what can assist, and some suggestions below have worked for me:

• take a cold shower, followed by warm water;

• make a hot cup of cocoa with honey and cinnamon to sip;

- concentrate on your breath – breathe normally and after an out breath, breathe in through your nose to your solar plexus and then slowly breathe out through your mouth, to form a kissing shape with puckered lips, repeat this as many times as you can with your mind focussing only on each breath and the next breath and soon you will fall asleep. It is vital to still the mind and focus only on the breathing;

- lavender oil is great to have near your pillow as it is calming and soothing; and

- keep a notebook and pen beside the bed to jot down what is on your mind.

Sometimes dreams can wake us – writing down what we have dreamed gets it out of our mind and then we can read later in the morning: often we forget the details if we go back to sleep. Writing down those little gems which woke us up helps us to clear the clutter from our head. Once on paper, it removes the challenge to remember these items.

A healthy lifestyle takes only a moment to plan – yet it is the execution that often derails us. I may have great intentions, yet the hectic pace of life sometimes impacts my practical everyday habits. Changing a habit does take approximately twenty-one to twenty-eight days – it depends on whose book you read – yet it is achievable. Changing a habit or introducing a habit is making a small change each day and then repeat, repeat, repeat. Words are easy to write, yet taking the time to make the daily modification can be life changing. I know that I love to take sunrise walks, and it takes discipline to ensure I get up that little bit earlier to fit in this exercise. These walks occur at least three times a week. Some habits are not necessarily daily, although they are part of a regular program.

Gaining vitality in this chapter combines many health aspects: mental health, physical health, nutrition, emotional wellbeing and spiritual awareness. Yet what is missing? Where is the joy in your life? Where is the fun in your life? What brings you joy? To me, many things bring me joy – spending time with my family, cooking for my family and friends, growing my herbs and veggies, and I love to dance. These activities are entwined in my life because I feel so beautiful inside. My heart sings. I have fun with these activities as often it sparks my creativity – through a new recipe, learning a new dance routine or finding a different plant to grow. Laughter is great medicine. And I often have a good belly laugh, either watching TV or reading a book.

Fun is different for all of us – yet spending time with people whose company brings smiles, laughter and good conversation can be great for the soul. Fun could be doing a crossword or doing a long bike ride or... *Your choice!* We have the power to choose joy and fun in our life. Each one of us has the ability to change the lens we look through and see the good in any situation. Experiencing and appreciating what brings you joy is paramount to having vitality. Reflect and decide; what do you want to change? If you have a block and feel resistant to shifting from a belief system that holds back your joy, write out an 11 x 22 with these words: "I am expressing myself perfectly..."

I like this quote from Steve Jobs, Co-founder and Chairman of CEO Apple Corporation, who passed in 2011 and just before his death, wrote an article about what is essential in life. He noted that although he was a billionaire, whether he had a watch worth $300 or $30 was irrelevant towards the end of his life. He further stated that how much you have earned may give you lots of trappings, yet taking time with family and friends to chat, laugh, sing songs and play games is paramount to achieving happiness. Cherish others. He makes a bold statement: *'Eat your food as your medicine; otherwise, you have to eat medicine as your food.'*[18] The famous quote below, often attributed to Hippocrates, talks to me about how nature and the

---

18 https://medium.com/oniverse/steve-jobs-last-words-e17b381a192e

simple things in life are of utmost importance to staying healthy:

'The six best doctors in the world are sunlight, rest,
exercise, diet, self- confidence and friends.
Maintain them in all stages and enjoy a healthy life.'

Are you ready to make some changes in your life? I have prepared **Action Aces** to help highlight the tools offered in this chapter and the summary to commence on one aspect right away. If you have it all together, fantastic!

Action Aces

▶ On an empty stomach, commence the day with three sticks of celery, washed and juiced. (Start with celery if you're doing both celery and lemon).

▶ Commence the day with the juice of half a freshly-squeezed lemon in a cup of hot water. Allow thirty minutes before you consume food and tea or coffee.

▶ Focus on your breath – whenever you wish to still the mind and bring calmness – slowly exhale before starting to breathe the sequences 3, 2, 5 or 4, 4, 4.

▶ Start morning shower with cold water for 10 seconds minimum. If you do not want to get your hair wet, ensure water runs between the brow and nape of the neck. Wet the front and back of your body as well with cold water.

▶ Are you okay? Know the conversation for yourself and to help others:

 • *'I've noticed that you haven't been yourself lately, is everything okay with you?'*[19]

 • *'I'm concerned about you. I'm wondering if we can talk about what's troubling you? You've seemed really down... sad... angry... unhappy lately. I'm worried that you might be thinking of hurting yourself or suicide. Can we talk about this?'*

▶ Utilise the de-cording exercise to energetically clear the emotions for three consecutive days and as required.

▶ Prepare a weekly menu to include fresh fruit and vegetables Introduce some exercise into your daily and weekly schedule.

▶ Drink one to two litres room temperature water per day.

▶ Sunshine exposure – enjoy natural Vitamin D.

---

19 Mindstar.com.au, 2019, *Suicide-Prevention*

▶ Clear the subconscious with 11 x 22s exercise – eleven consecutive days with positive "I" sentences to release distorted energy. Write sentence twenty-two times with whatever thought pops into your mind after the positive start. Do not re-read your sentences. Discard the written words daily.

For example:

1. I am well and healthy *in every moment.*

2. I am well and healthy *when I'm feeling lost and unmotivated.*

Sentence for Illness:

My... (whichever part of the body is causing a problem)
is perfect and clear...

Sentence for Joy:

I am expressing myself perfectly...

Clearing Your Subconscious 11 x 22s:

- *The subconscious is stored within our cells.*

- *The process of using numbers with repeated affirmative sentences can break down a belief pattern.*

- *On an energetic level, the positive words enter into the mind and body, pushing out distorted energy.*

- *An internal shift then occurs as the distortion is dispersed through the aura, leaving it clear.*

▶ Have a pen and paper beside your bed to write down information gems during night hours.

- Ensure you have a good sleep routine to keep you vital and happy.

- List the activities that bring you absolute joy and make sure they are part of your daily and weekly routine.

Oil Pulling Technique[20]

1. In the morning on an empty stomach and before drinking any liquids, take one tablespoon of oil into your mouth. If you do this in the evening, it MUST be on an empty stomach.

2. Swish the oil around in your mouth without swallowing it. Move it around and through your teeth, similar to using a mouthwash. DO NOT GARGLE IT. You will find that the oil starts to get watery as your saliva mixes with it. Keep swishing it around. If your jaw muscles ache, you are doing it too hard. Relax the jaw muscles. Use the tongue to help you to move the liquid around the inside of your mouth. Do this for approximately twenty minutes.

3. If you have the unbearable urge to swallow, vomit, or if it becomes too unpleasant, spit it out and try again. It may take a few attempts before getting used to having oil in your mouth. At approximately the twenty minutes mark, spit the oil out into a glass and rinse the mouth with water. It is also beneficial to brush your teeth.

4. A good indication of detoxification is if the oil is white or milky in colour. If it has remained the yellow of oil colour, you will need to do the twenty minutes session again. The milky white consistency is proof of toxic elimination in the saliva.

5. Repeat process for seven days minimum to experience the benefits.

---

20 Jo Le Rose, *Healthy Atom Detox Program worksheet*, 7 January 2014

CHAPTER THREE

Feeling Fear
– Gaining Courage

*"Remember: nothing is ever a failure, it is just
a lesson learned, to do things another way."*

Karen Nelson

I have experienced fear. I was stopped in my tracks – immobilised.
I procrastinated because I did not want to put myself out there.
I was scared of what others may think. Once I took the plunge
and something went wrong, I would beat myself up for days or
weeks and in my mind, it was like a tortuous video on continuous
replay. I questioned why I participated in the first place? Have you
experienced these signs and symptoms of fear?

Many setbacks gave me the courage to learn and grow – though
they were very painful at the time – and even from a young age
I would want to improve on my knowledge and through this I
developed courage to have another go. It is important to remember
that when things go wrong, we get results. I use the adage that every
cloud has a silver lining and I always look for the shine of silver in
every situation. Sometimes it is not the result I had expected, yet it
allowed me to look to my role in the situation and what could I have
done differently.

Next time when something does not go to plan, write down three
things you discovered, learned or perhaps a benefit which emerged

from the mistake. Alternatively, write down what you would do differently next time if you are presented with a similar situation.

The great educator and scientist George Washington Carver said, *"Ninety-nine per cent of failures come from people who have a habit of making excuses."* Remember, opportunity is a visitor: don't assume it will be back tomorrow. *Now* is the time – move while the door is open![21]

What's making you hesitate?

I have experienced physical and psychological fear during my life; maybe you have as well.

Physical fear is often referred to as the fight-or-flight response and is an instinct. If you find yourself in a perceived threatening situation in response to acute stress, the body's sympathetic nervous system becomes activated due to a quick release of hormones that stimulate the adrenal glands, triggering a release of adrenaline and noradrenaline. Once the danger passes, the body regulates itself. The fight response gives you the stamina to stay and defend the situation, whereas the flight response tells you to run and get away from the threat.

Psychological fear is when our mind delivers all kinds of scenarios about people and situations, causing the mind to be concerned, resulting in worry about the unknown consequence. This type of fear impacts us significantly as we are often worried about what other people say or think about us. Just consider if you stopped and thought about a belief that was told to you as a child – sometime in your formative years of zero to seven – and if you reviewed it and challenged in your mind as to whether it was true or false. I remember repeatedly hearing that *'Children should be seen and not heard.'* It impacted me for a good number of years as I would often

---

21 https://vision.org.au/the-word-for-today/associated-blog/the-word-fortoday-devotional-content/move-while-the-door-is-open/ Bob and Debby Gass, *The Word for Today*, Tuesday 14 May 2019

not speak up, as this belief was implanted firmly in my psyche. No doubt, my mother heard this from her mother. Consequently, my sister and I were raised on this belief which conditioned our mind for a very long time. Luckily, we have changed. We did not raise our children on this belief; we broke the conditioning cycle.

What I do know about fear is that it leaves you powerless... do you agree? Feeling powerless is the root of fear. The feelings of being inadequate, lacking courage, not getting it *right*, scared to take the next step because failure is so humiliating, and we would rather live this small life because it is supposedly *safe*. Physically and emotionally, we are without power.

A couple of years ago, I spent time with a client who felt she was not being paid the correct Industrial Award amount for her position. I researched and deduced that her annualised salary was indeed below the hourly rate for that position. Therefore, she was being short-changed about $3,000-odd in her wage. It can quickly occur when a company does not look at the yearly Consumer Price Index (CPI) increase on the hourly rate and multiply it out to find the difference for an annualised salary. After discussions, I prepared a letter for her, and we registered this issue with the relevant authority. My client went away with a note for the company and shared this information with her dad. Her dad said that she would lose her job if she raised this issue, and it was better to have a job than highlighting the inequity. This lovely lady heeded the words of her father. His beliefs were so strong that she felt compelled to accept them, and yes, not having a job would impact her financially. This story highlights the dad's beliefs and fears which he passed onto his daughter.

Often during my formative years, my mind took on the belief that I needed to struggle through life. You may have heard people say things like 'We need to have some setbacks as this makes us strong.' I remember repeating this. Our mind is so powerful, yet we still believe something we took on as a child of less than seven years old. It is timely to revisit old beliefs and allocate a timeframe to sit with what is concerning you. To understand and get clear about the beginnings of that belief. For some people, it will take several sessions of sitting with the idea. For others who have been pondering their thoughts and feelings, it may take a short time. There is no right or wrong. To help yourself, allow some quiet time to reflect and **feel** the emotion and discover where it originated. Sometimes feeling the emotion will bring a physical change where the heart might palpitate, the stomach might tighten and churn, the eyes will shed tears, or even laughter breaks out as a release. Ask yourself, is this truly my belief today?

Let's change our focus to living in power and being limitless! You can change by exploring the belief and dispelling it as it is not what you currently believe, yet subconsciously you are still carrying the theory from your childhood. We came into this earth to have fun and to bring joy. I remember working on an international project and telling the management team that we are here to have fun! Wow – that caused a reaction. We spend so much time at work, and it is imperative to enjoy what you do and have fun doing it. I hope you will explore and gain a better understanding of what your purpose is on earth, and asking; does it bring joy to your life?

I have observed through life that if I focus on being abundant, that I genuinely *am* abundant in every aspect. Conversely, if I focus on the negative point of being in lack – then I am in lack in every way. What we focus on is what we draw towards us and ultimately experience. Our thoughts lead to feelings. What we feel has a lot to do with how we live our life. Feeling into the energy of abundance, for example, allows for many blessings to flow. I have food to eat, shelter for each night, clothes to wear, money to cover my expenses, good health allowing exercise, and I have amazing like-minded friends. When I am in this feeling, I have high vibrations, and I feel good! Alternatively, when fear takes hold of me, I have low vibrations. During one of my courses I learned about fear's opposite, love. We were asked to look at our own emotions and examine what we experience between the emotion of fear and love. As I compiled a set of my emotional scales it reminded me of a vivid painting at a Patmos Church in Greece, where the painting depicted Jacob's dream where he saw a stairway resting on the earth and reaching to heaven.[22] The artwork was fairly graphic with people falling into pits with serpents and it reminded me of how I experienced fear and went into a negative place – maybe not necessarily with snakes – yet definitely into a dark part of myself. Conversely, the upside of the painting illustrated the house of God and the gate of heaven, which to me reflected pure, unconditional love and freedom.

1. *Love/Freedom*
2. *Joy/Appreciation*
3. *Passion*
4. *Happiness*
5. *Excitement*
6. *Optimism*
7. *Contentment*
8. *Hope*
9. *Withdrawal*
10. *Frustration*
11. *Disappointment*
12. *Blame*
13. *Irritation*
14. *Jealousy*
15. *Anger*
16. *Guilt*
17. *Despair*
18. *Unworthiness*
19. *Fear/Powerless*

---

22 Genesis 28: vs10–19, *The NIV Study Bible*

My ladder of emotions as it scales through the various emotions that represent me.

The numbers on the left-hand side give an indication of the highest priority, commencing at one and moving through to nineteen. What is important to note is that these emotions are indicators of my vibrational frequency and that I choose to keep my vibrations in a range of one to six. Not always of course. Through choice, the better I feel, then the more that I am allowing the alignment of things that I desire. As an example, when I am in that alignment range, I feel free, I feel purpose; I am love and I have value. It is like having fuel in my car and there is an indicator advising if I am running on full, on empty, or in between. And so, it is similar with the indicators of my emotions, not naming the emotion per se; it's more about how I am feeling overall and whether that feeling has improved. In essence, when I'm running on full, I have a great connection with myself and source energy, and when I'm on empty I am showing resistance within myself and my source energy.

You might find it useful to write your ladder of emotional scales and understand where you emotionally spend the most time. When I indicate love / freedom I am speaking about pure love – unconditional love, which is different to romantic love. At a time in my life when I loved someone, there was an underlying belief that 'Because I do this for you, then you will love me for doing that,' and also vice versa. That is not unconditional love, which evolves where there is no judgement and I do a task seeking nothing in return – it is true freedom for the people who exchange unconditional love.

Reading the book 'When things fall apart', by Pema Chodron, there is a story about a Tibetan man who learns how to face fear, and his teacher provides stories which assist with his growth, plus examples of courage when facing fear.[23] One story particularly stayed with me, and that was about travelling to a monastery he'd

---

23 Pema Chodron, *When things fall apart*, p22

never been before. As the group approached the gates, a ferocious guard dog snarled at them and tried to free itself from the chain. They managed to walk past the dog and entered the gate. All of a sudden the chain broke, and the dog rushed at the group. Others in the group screamed and ran away. The Tibetan man, however, turned and ran as fast as he could – straight at the dog. The dog was so surprised that he scampered away with its tail between his legs. Each of us have one of a fight or flight response. Some in the group froze in terror. Some ran. The Tibetan man's heart opened and brought forth courage. I found this a compelling story of facing fear and gaining courage.

Some of my fears are shared with you so that you can find the answers within, and have the courage to take the first step to change with the help of tools I have used. Taking the first step is always the hardest. Chat to a close friend who will support you and also hold you to account.

Fear of failure
Lose the fear of failing

We can't make progress without failing.
Fear of failing holds us back.
Most successful people fail more often than they succeed,
But they persist.
Failing is just improving your chances of succeeding next time.
Allow yourself the possibility of failing.

Patrick Lindsay

At one stage my life was topsy-turvy with several changes of address, a change of jobs through redundancy and a study opportunity. For a long time, I always wanted to attend university and as circumstances unfolded, the timing was opening to this dream. Nevertheless, I had to trust myself that all the signs were pointing to this. I worked on a project that finished prematurely and while I continued employment in the Human Resources field for this particular company, there was a definite feel that my role would cease, allowing university attendance for one full-time year of study. I was hesitant in taking the next step as I had not completed grade twelve: I finished at grade ten and attended secretarial college, like many women during that time had done. While I held diploma qualifications, I was not sure whether I would be accepted, yet I applied and anxiously awaited news of my progression. I received correspondence for an interview at the university for a place to undertake a Master of Human Resource Management. I was terrified that I would fail.

Have you ever had those feelings of being so nervous that it impacts your voice projection? When your nervousness affects your bladder, requiring numerous trips to the bathroom? Somehow the goal of wanting to attend this course allowed me to project my voice and despite being visibly nervous, the panel could see I had loads of experience as indicated on my resume, and they advised that I would be accepted. In my recruitment world, we often say that if a person has twenty years of experience (in their chosen field), then that equates to a bachelor's degree.

I was thrilled and at the same time, anxious – how would I go? My biggest fear at the time was the fear of failure. Have you ever wanted something *so badly*, yet kept putting off the inevitable because of that niggling feeling inside your head, that just kept playing out all the negatives about failure, loss of face, and that you weren't good enough?

I had previously completed lots of short courses which gave me the relevant qualifications, along with a wealth of knowledge. I have a saying that *'When all the doors open, it is meant to be!'* Well, this time all the doors opened! I felt I was ready to take a chance –

a chance on me. What did I have to lose? The considerable cost of the degree, of course, yet more than that, I would have to tell family and friends of my failure. If I didn't pass all the subjects, there was always a chance to select another topic or repeat it. That might hurt my pride: yet I did have options.

The positives outweighed the negatives, and I reminded myself that many great people have failed and kept going. We know them now as icons – think Albert Einstein, Katy Perry, Oprah Winfrey, J.K. Rowling, Bill Gates, Stephen King and Henry Ford, to name just a few. Indeed, when the people I listed here failed, the one thing they all had in common was the ability to keep going. They had a **vision**. Each had a **goal** and **courage** reigned.

What does it mean to have a vision?

To me, it is the goal that I want to reach within a specific timeframe. It is future paced using the present tense: I will attend university and obtain a Master of Human Resource Management degree within twelve months. Having a good vision inspired and energised me and provided a vivid mental picture of what it will look like at the end of the period. I visualised myself proudly wearing the cap and gown at the graduation ceremony with family and close friends sharing my celebration.

What does it mean to have a goal?

'An observable and measurable end result having one or more objectives, to be achieved within a more or less fixed timeframe.'[24] Yes, I had a goal that I would measure each semester, and my objective was to obtain a Credit score or above successfully on all subjects within the twelve month timeframe.

---

24 http://www.businessdictionary.com/definition/goal.html

There is another aspect to goal setting: based on whether you are motivated by wanting to achieve a positive outcome or avoid an adverse one. My goal was considered an 'approach goal'. Dr Susan Peppercorn wrote in a Harvard Business Review article that psychologists have found that positively reframing avoidance goals is beneficial for wellbeing.[25] Sometimes when you are dealing with difficult or distasteful tasks, you may unconsciously set goals around what you don't want to happen rather than what you do want. Focusing on what you want to achieve is far more beneficial than setting an avoidance goal. It is a subtle line of difference – take the time to review how you perceive the outcome. Avoidance goals are a common approach to perceived failure, and statistically, it shows that people who take this approach are twice as mentally fatigued as those who take on the approach goal mindset. When I removed my focus from potential failure to 'What could I learn from undertaking this level of study?' I embraced each subject as bringing me towards the ultimate goal of attaining the degree. With my first subject, I received a Credit, and while it was higher than a Pass, I wanted a better result. My reaction could have gone two ways – I'm not good enough, and disappointment that that was all that I received in marks – or I could decide that I would learn from this and improve for next assignment. I chose the approach goal rather than the avoidance goal, read the lecturer's notes carefully and made changes in how I put my argument in the next assignment, achieving a result of Distinction.

What does it mean to have courage?

I wanted to have courage – I read stories from a very young age about David battling Goliath in the Bible story, the Cowardly Lion in the Wizard of Oz who finds the courage to face the witch – as children we were raised habitually on these and similar stories. We often think of physical courage, yet it is often more than that. Many

---

25 https://hbr.org/2018/12/how-to-overcome-your-fear-of-failure

prominent people speak out about injustice at high personal risk, illustrating the adage to have the courage of your convictions. It is a brave person who realises that it takes courage to feel triumph over fear. A quote that resonates is from Steve Jobs' Stanford commencement speech, in June 2005. *'And most important, have the courage to follow your heart and intuition. They somehow know what you truly want to become. Everything else is secondary.'* To me, this aligns with a passion for doing something – it is the driver that gave me the courage to take that leap. My leap was having the courage to expand my horizon – learning more and obtaining a recognised degree. I faced studying full on and gave it my all, in order to obtain my dream of higher education.

At first, it was tough. Not knowing anyone studying the course and being a mature age student, I felt out of place. I observed the campus grounds, and there were lots of people of all ages and demographics – this helped me realise that at any age, people study. I took opportunities and attended all free lectures on assignment writing and assessment preparation. I extended myself further out of my comfort zone. I selected a subject of statistics – a real challenge at a master's level – to further broaden my prospects of employment once I'd finished the study. I spent many hours researching, writing and re-writing and weekends at the university. Subjects required up to date data from within the last two years, and online research and international journals provided interesting articles for discussion and debate. Group work was a challenge, with two to four people having a set of objectives to achieve within a determined timeframe, and the marks were equal for all – whether one or all four contributed. Now I fully realised that this was just like paid work, with small groups of people coming together to fulfil a task. As I realigned the study to work environments, part of me relaxed and faced the fear as I drew on my considerable workplace experience.

I learned that by taking action, there is a visible consequence. By taking action each day, no matter how small or large, I was facing my fear in bite-sized pieces. The doing – my action – was critical. I found a quote when reading Stephen R Covey's 1997 book, 'The 7 Habits of Highly Effective Families', in which he quotes Viktor E. Frankl that became a silent reminder:

'Between stimulus and response, there is a space. In that space lies our freedom and power to choose our response. In our response lies our growth and our happiness.'

I printed out this quote and have it to this day, because it is a constant reminder that I have a choice – and now, so do you. You currently have an opportunity to take action to face your fear and gain courage. I faced my fear and succeeded with flying colours. It certainly had times of tears, tiredness and dogged determination, yet each time I took action there was a visible consequence. I learned so much about myself during this time, and not only from an academic aspect, for example, I found that I could get very nervous when I had to speak in front of lecturers and my peers, which now is not a concern. I learned that even though some subjects were stretching me, maybe too thin, it was me who was in control of how I faced that stretch and my outlook was a key motivator as well as strength during these challenges. I dug deep to find the courage to face the opportunities – they may have felt like challenges, yet I chose to consider them as opportunities for growth. Courage is facing the fear head-on, and I was gaining confidence with each opportunity. I received the award of Academic Excellence for my second semester efforts, which filled my heart with gratitude plus a quiet sense of achievement.

Fear of shame

"Have fun, fail fast and forgive yourself."

Yvette Luciano

I travelled overseas to attend a course in Israel, where I stayed near the Dead Sea on a kibbutz. The kibbutz is a cooperative community, usually self-supporting with growing their foods, and each family supports the commune with their skills and talents. We shared accommodation with others on the course, and we ate in the kibbutz dining areas and observed and joined with their activities at night, such as traditional dancing.

Towards the end of the course, I signed up for a horse-riding activity. From an early age, I had a belief that I had a 'hot seat' as when I sat on a horse, it took off – to my horror. I enjoyed viewing horses from afar, as my Godparents Keith and Elsie had a lovely horse named Valentine. I was too scared to feed her carrots and nearly dropped the carrot during times that I tried. Yes, my fear of failure in this instance was a fear of shame.

The day arrived for the horse-riding activity in the kibbutz. I imagined a stroll around the boundary of the enclosed corral and felt that it would be manageable. Before setting foot into the paddock, I actually had nervous diarrhoea; I was anxious beyond belief. I received assistance to mount the horse and then I contemplated not going through with this venture as I could not cope. I removed the camera from around my neck as I couldn't focus on holding the reins and trying to capture the view from the horse. I was just too nervous.

I thought if I stay on just a few moments longer, then I can get off! I was torn between escaping from this self-imposed adventure or actually facing my fear and just doing it. We were given commands in Arabic for the horse and told some simple techniques for using the reins. Okay, I can do this! No, I want to run away! Let me escape as this is too hard to face. The thoughts vacillated in my head from *'Get off now!'* to *'You can do it.'* The inner turmoil was intense.

To my relief, a friend who is an excellent horsewoman and worked at the kibbutz rode alongside me, providing support, comfort and coaxing words. I knew that no-one could do this for me; I had to face this challenge. I was blessed to have Alexandra's support. Those very close to me knew of my anxiety. We set off on a ride through the date plantation – up hills and down gullies, pebbles, rocks, diversions – and fear gripped me. At the best of times, I sometimes get my left and right muddled, yet my frazzled brain couldn't cope on this occasion. My mare of some twenty-eight years knew the route and provided me with confidence. Although we were the last in the group, I slowly relaxed and observed the scenery that surrounded us: rows upon rows of date trees and the tranquillity of just being in nature. We were lagging; my mare suddenly cantered to reach the others. My heart jumped! It was another leap of faith to stay on and somehow enjoy this moment of freedom amongst my jarred nerves.

After what seemed ages, although in reality it was probably thirty minutes, we all stopped for a break and ate dates freshly picked from the tree. Wow, sensational. Photos duly taken, and after several minutes we were trekking on our homeward journey. I relaxed a little more, realising I'd made it so far and there was only half an hour more. The wonderful mare knew the route so my commands and turning the reins, while necessary, were not vital as she just followed the twenty or so horses returning. My joy and happiness upon reaching the stables overflowed. As I dismounted – with help – my legs felt bowed, yet my heart sang with joy. I did it! I completed my horse ride.

The horse-riding experience allowed me to persevere in the face of adversity. Yes, I was afraid beyond belief, yet the inner voice wanted me to succeed despite my perceived danger. I feel that J. R. R. Tolkien, writing in 'The Hobbit' sums up my feelings beautifully:

"Go back?" he thought. "No good at all! Go sideways? Impossible! Go forward? The only thing to do! On we go!" So up he got and trotted along with his little sword held in front of him and one hand feeling the wall, and his heart all of a patter and a pitter."

That night in the kibbutz, we enjoyed a campfire with music and dancing. My smile was wide, my heart free, and I danced with such abandonment and freedom and pure joy. What a celebration evening – not only had I conquered my fear of horses, I had unlocked a new part of me that touches and impacts other areas of my life.

Have you ever felt terrified to undertake a task? Have you felt the immobilisation to the point of doing nothing? It can creep in and blindside you. Panic sets in and fear raises its ugly visage. These are the characteristics that fear takes on in our mind, which then flows to our physical body. Fear can be paralysing. It can turn our life around – if we let it. We do have power over our minds and how we decide to use that fear to our highest good. There is a choice that we can make – taking action each day to achieve our vision and goal will assist with the desired result. Consistency in taking action to face the fear is the key to overcoming it. Some of us take large bites, and some of us take a nibble. Neither is right nor wrong. It is taking the bite, large or small, which is critical.

Fear of success

"Success for the sake of success does not lead to soul fulfilment."

Yvette Luciano

There have been times in my life when I visualised my expansion, and it scared me. Fear of my success was genuine, as I was afraid that my depth and breadth of success could be considerable. A portion of me wanted to shut down this aspect as in my mind it grew larger than life. It felt as though I could scale a mountain and reach the top, imbued with energy and enthusiasm. In Australia, we have what is commonly named *'tall poppy syndrome'*, meaning jealousy of someone who excels or achieves more than others, and Australians like to cut down *'tall poppies'*. Perhaps culturally, I didn't want to be that tall poppy blowing in the breeze, reaching the sky and achieving goals. Yet, another part of me wanted to bask in the achievement limelight of inner knowing. I do hope that as our nation's history grows, we will salute those who succeed and honour the vision of the many people who are labelled *'tall poppies'*. Remember, it is only a label and not one that you have to accept nor follow that belief. A lesson to me for sure.

This fear of success had been on a sub-conscious level for a long time, and more recently, I have found a strength within me to embrace all that I am. Working through this fear, I spent many hours in nature. Being at the beach or in a rainforest or a bush environment allows me to listen to the birds and other sounds, to view the ground I walk upon and to see the fantastic colours and textures and to just be in that moment with nature. Because I love nature, my inner child comes out to explore and I'm excited to see a rainbow, to find a shell, to see a seagull, to identify a tree specimen and enjoy the flowers or the shape of a leaf, to smell the freshness of a lemon-scented gum or breathe in the saltwater air. These small things light up my face and I smile; there is a warm feeling within me which I label as joyous. You are probably wondering how does this help? Well, each of us has an inner being or inner compass or intuition. We may call it different things, yet it shows our signposts in life, directing us on our path. Our intuition does not know right or wrong: it just knows ' it is'. Building our intuition is about taking time in nature to appreciate the sounds, the smells, the sights, the feelings and to be aware of touch. It stills my mind as I appreciate what is all around me. Not everyone is blessed with these surroundings, yet when I am away, I visualise a picture (real or imaginary) to take myself to this happy place in my mind.

THE ANSWERS ARE WITHIN

At a workshop early in my journey of self-discovery, Mike Robinson taught an excellent tool to help us decipher what our intuition is saying to us. Do you know that each of us has an energy field around us? This field is our natural chi. If you were to ask yourself a simple question which has a "yes" or "no" response, you could use your chi to assist the answer. Stand with your legs slightly apart, ask the question and notice if your chi energy moves somewhat forward or slightly backward. If your body sways forward, it is acknowledging a "yes", and if it pulls you slightly back, it is answering "no". I have built up this strength, and it is vital to spend time recharging in nature so that we can feel the changes around us and within us. Others have expressed that I am very grounded – perhaps this is a result of my time in nature and doing my inner compass observations. I also utilise visualisations and take time to meditate. Meditation takes many forms and just spending time in nature and observing can be classified as meditating. Equally, chanting and repeating mantras is also a form of meditation. Meditation allows us to go within to find our inner guidance. It is a time to have peace and inner knowing, which assists our overall good health.

Matthieu Ricard, an author and Buddhist monk, states that *'The object of meditation is the mind.'*[26] His reflections observe that the mind is not shut down during meditation, instead meditation assists it to be *'free, lucid and balanced.'* He further states that it requires time to train the mind to refine and sharpen our attention, develop emotional balance and inner peace. My way of describing this would be to build the muscle of the mind by taking the time to watch our thoughts. Take time to remove the ego; become observant to inner freedom, let go of limitations and hardships and set one's course. As I evolve, I find giving myself time to just breathe in and breathe out, as stilling the mind gives alignment to my source and providing that I let go of any resistance, I feel such peace and joy in my being. Feel your thoughts (ideas, dreams) come into words and

---

26 Matthieu Ricard, *The Art of Meditation*, p29–33

allow for the journey to unfold during this time of inner reflection. You become what you immerse yourself in – therefore if you take meditation time, you become calm and centred. If you watch television endlessly, then you absorb what you watch. Experiment for yourself.

I also love playing music to assist with a meditative state. Bach music is calming and cleansing. If you have not listened to this classical composer, give it a try. Bach's baroque music matches the beat of the heart. As I write, I have Bach's CD playing, and it is the Brandenburg Concertos 2-3-5 by the Amsterdam Festival Orchestra. Johann Bach was a German composer and musician during the Baroque period, who was born in 1685 and died in 1750 aged 65 years. He studied intensely and drew on well-known composers of his time and then added his stamp. One of my favourites is Toccata and Fugue in D minor for violins.

You may enjoy taking some time to explore an expansive visualisation. Sit in an open space, preferably with lots of space – try a park or the beach – and start an expansion of yourself. Extending out to the area where you are sitting, then further around you in the park or beach, and then beyond. Go further, again expanding to the horizon and even further to encompass the planet. You are limitless! Keep this visualisation regularly occurring, as it will diminish the fear, and the positive vibes will attract that expansive success to you like a magnet.

There are times when I have used fast writing to empty the thoughts in my mind onto paper. It is an easy way to release the fear by just writing out what pops into my head and then disposing of it via burning the paper or soaking in cold water. Of course, I have also done 11 x 22s as outlined in this chapter's **Action Aces**. I certainly did a variation which is three days with the sentence written seventy-five times. Allow plenty of time allocation to achieve this in three days, as the same rules apply in that it must be three consecutive days.

Sometimes if I am thinking of someone, then that is where my energy flows. This book is predominately about me (and you) and therefore I want my energy to be with me. If I want to break that energy attachment, I have found a visualisation exercise of closing seven doors most successful. Instructions are in the **Action Aces**. My stories may or may not resonate with you, yet it's imperative that you take action, especially when fear is high.

Once you start facing your fear, you may wonder why you didn't commence sooner! Get started with the prompts in **Action Aces**.

Action Aces

Recognise what fear is holding you back.

Fear of failure, fear of shame,
fear of success, fear of looking foolish,
fear of not meeting another's expectations,
fear of doing something wrong, fear of...

Write down your fear's checklist:
(what you are afraid to do and what will happen if you do it)

Redefine the failure:

▶ Allow your mindset to look at the external factors over which you have no control. *E.g. the university only has six places for mature students, and 12 have applied.*

▶ What is failure? *E.g. not submitting any assignments; not applying to do the course.*

▶ What small results will give you success? *E.g. passing one subject at a time.*

▶ What does success look like, feel like? *E.g. finishing the degree with flying colours. Relief! Accomplishment!*

▶ What quote will you select for courage? Apply your definition of courage ...

▶ Identify the person with whom you can discuss the situation and share your feelings in a confidential capacity or seek professional help through a qualified coach.

▶ What support do you need to take the next step? When will you take the next step?

▶ How will you feel when you face your fear?

▶ What have you observed about the inner you and nature?

- ▶ What else?
- ▶ How will you celebrate your achievement?
- ▶ What gems have you gained that will help others and assist you to progress further?
  - *Emotional scales – make your own, so you know where you sit at any time*
  - *Listen to Bach music and appreciate the calming and cleansing effects*
  - *Clear the subconscious with 11 x 22s exercise – eleven consecutive days with positive "I" sentences to release distorted energy. Write your sentence twenty-two times with whatever thought pops into your mind after the positive start. Do not re-read your sentences. Discard the written words daily.*

For example:

1. I have the courage to achieve all that I desire *in each moment.*
2. I have the courage to achieve all that I desire *when I'm feeling lost and confused.*

Another Sentence for Fear: **Life is perfect right now...**

Clearing Your Subconscious 11 x 22s:

- *The subconscious is stored within our cells.*
- *The process of using numbers with repeated affirmative sentences can break down a belief pattern.*
- *On an energetic level, the positive words enter into the mind and body, pushing out distorted energy.*
- *An internal shift then occurs as the distortion is dispersed through the aura, leaving it clear.*

- ▶ Write down all that is currently going on to release many thoughts onto paper – known as fast writing. Do not read – discard.

- ▶ Visualisation – Closing the Seven Doors:

  - *When you are thinking of someone just visualise wherever they are and imagine there are seven doors – it can be in a tunnel, it can be seven doors around you, your mind in a circle if you like, all seven doors, or it might be a corridor and you just shut the seven doors.*

  - *The actual act of doing that shuts your energy down and breaks the connection, so you are still connected but you are not connected through that mental plane and the astral plane.*

  - *The doors may come to you as wooden doors – you might feel that one of them is a big, safe door. There might be metal doors – however it comes to you – when you think of that person, if you find them, just shut the seven doors and do it in your mind, simply see them in your inner mind.*

CHAPTER FOUR

Feeling Unworthy – Gaining Acceptance

"There is no blame, just lessons:
Stop right now and take a good look at yourself, dear one.
Summon courage and step back and observe your life.
How you feel, behave, how you think.
What part of you needs changing, needs pruning?
Who or what do you need to let go?
Do not deviate from your endeavour to discover your true self.
Take time to ask yourself who you are and what is your
purpose in this lifetime?
Acceptance lies within, within the heart of God.
Only in this sacred place lies true peace and happiness."

Patricia L Dryden, *Soul Poems of Love*

Let's get clear on the meaning of unworthy: the dictionary defines it as not deserving respect or attention, not acceptable and having little merit. Can you relate to those words?

Emotionally when I feel unworthy there is the little girl inside of me who feels very small – someone who feels she never measures up; not included in clique groups. I remember attending a 'Back to School' themed dinner and borrowed someone's school tie and badges. One lady at the function said to me, 'You never attended that private school – why are you wearing the uniform?' I brushed her comments aside, yet I felt unsettled as I didn't belong in that exclusive circle held together with school bonds. Luckily, I was in my thirties and it didn't define who I was then.

Sometimes I have felt as though my best was not good enough. Things like swimming – I love the water although I am not a strong swimmer of any distance. At school, it was compulsory to attend swimming carnivals, and students were encouraged to participate – maybe 'forced' is a better descriptor – in swimming 50 metres freestyle. Towards the end, I was struggling. I was gulping water. Swimming squad members were ready to jump in and save me and I felt humiliated as I wanted to be accepted as a cool teenager. Learning to swim lessons in my early years involved being pushed into the pool and shouted at when I didn't get things right. Those hurtful memories returned at the swimming carnival. I was not good enough to join the swimming squad, and the feelings of being unworthy came flooding back. My pain was deep. Have you experienced times of not fitting into a sport or similar event? Did you experience the feelings that hamper progress?

I have found that unworthiness shows up internally and externally. Internally it can be the negative self-talk – the chatter and thoughts inside my mind leading to a low vibration. It seemed like things went astray and I felt not worthy to receive that promotion, or not deserving of that loving relationship or that my education did not reach the desired level to progress my career. Internally was the feeling that I had attracted these situations and upon self-observation, the conclusion was that I was negative and in low vibration.

Externally, unworthiness is when others voice their opinions about me or my situation that sometimes can be a judgement. In my mind, I take on this opinion, and it continues the spiral. It is human to hear another's opinion; yet it is equally important to look at ourselves and feel into the words to see if they resonate with us, or is it actually a projection from the other person about themselves? Taking time to feel into the situation was paramount to understanding myself. I ask myself the question: *'Is this true about me?'* It became a time to be totally honest with myself, and the more I realised, yes, this is me, then the easier it became to accept the truth. The more I denied, then the inner work did not occur, and I continued on the cycle of not trusting my intuition. Through acceptance that I am not perfect, it was okay to feel this way. At times, it was not about me. It was about the other person's projections. The more that I got to know myself – warts and all – the easier it was to distinguish: is this about me or is it about them?

Gaining acceptance of myself was and is a continuing journey, not a judgement. I observed and accepted what I noticed about myself and sometimes others. It is okay to have different feelings or responses to a given situation, and while I may have preferred a better answer or result, that is all that I was capable of at the time. It is not a time to berate myself. It is not a time to continually repeat the situation. It was a reflective time to what has occurred within me and to find self-acceptance.

After gaining my degree and while actively seeking work, I met spiritual teacher Mike Robinson in Australia at the first week intensive of his course to complete a Certificate in Natural Healing. It was an extraordinary time for me as I discovered that I could actually *'see'* into my body and noticed the beautiful colours and organs. It was a moment of euphoria and also *'Did I just see that?'* An ah-ha moment. Profound times of inner work commenced, and these intensives gave me time to take action and implement many of the learnings. At different moments fear showed its ugly features, but I have learned to accept myself just as I am, at and in that moment. Learning to observe my feelings was a critical turning point and more importantly to actually *feel* the emotions it raised. It took continual access to what I was *feeling* and not what my head was saying – a mindset change. I would remind myself, *'Get out of your head and into your heart.'* I completed the exams for the Certificate of Natural Healing and felt that my journey was opening areas in my life that I never expected. Two years later, I did a refresher and completed the Advanced Counselling Certificate. This course has given me insight into the body, mind and soul of my being. It is a continuing journey of learning.

Before my university study, the project in which I worked closed down due to budget overruns. It is ironic that upon finishing my degree a blind advert appeared in a newspaper for an HR Officer and from the description of the position, I sensed that this was the project where I was previously employed. Correct. My previous employment was through a Joint Venture partner, and this time it was with the owner's team – absolutely ideal in a project environment. My application was successful, with commencement just after the Natural Healing residential course. It was a time when I believed in my skills and in a short time, I progressed to Human Resources Manager.

The Project Director, to whom I reported, was visionary and skilled with managing very large projects, and he provided the mentoring for me to keep progressing my skills. His belief in me also boosted my confidence, and soon there was a high-performance human resources team. The ladies in this team were enthusiastic and together we brainstormed heaps of ideas and made a significant difference to procedures to ensure that we remained financially viable, as well as providing the fun required to work in a fluid environment. I kept learning more about myself as a leader and manager as we gained acceptance from all parties on continuous change. I found that communication is a vital key in gaining acceptance. Chatting to our internal people and also our external suppliers was a priority to get buy-in on ideas as we all wanted the same result for project success. Having difficult conversations when required and being honest with communication builds trust. I found the management team to be of the highest quality and communication was open and honest, even when sharing opposing views on a topic. These endeavours strengthened the acceptance of the person as we understood their values; collectively, this contributed to better decision making with the alignment of the project's outcomes.

I travelled to Toronto, Canada, to meet the management personnel of the parent company and to familiarise myself with Human Resource policy and procedures. On my first journey to the office, I walked the footpaths huddled in multiple warm layers as the wind was biting. It was November and freezing cold. I had accepted that the way to the office was similar to life in Australia – just walk along the footpath to the intended destination. Luckily, the staff showed me how the locals made their way to work and I quickly took mental notes on the labyrinth of underground shopping centres and walkways, carefully noting where to turn so that I returned safely to my hotel. I was so thankful for these little gems of local information. I could have easily said 'I'm okay, I know the way,' as I followed the map. Yet my learning was to accept the offer of local knowledge as a better way to transverse the city and keep myself warm. Sometimes just showing up and being guided to listen to others can produce amazing results.

Working on a project is very fluid, and change occurs regularly within a project cycle. I enjoy change and accept and manage it quite well. For my personal life, I continued to attend courses that inspired and challenged my self-development. It has been quoted that one year in a project equals three years in the real job world. On many occasions, project management personnel worked fifty-five to sixty hours per week, plus additional travel time, as the project construction site was in New Caledonia. It certainly felt like ten years of work condensed into five years, as each phase of the project involved people finishing in their specialised roles – such as design – and then onto construction stage and finally into commissioning. Each aspect required a high level of skill and managers required processes that would monitor the timeframes and delivery methodologies. Each phase of the project was a separate section of work. Acceptance that projects have a start date and a finish date was not always easy.

You could imagine that part of finishing a project meant that each person had to start looking for alternative work. Seasoned project workers accepted that this was a chosen way of life and their higher rates of pay compensated for this phase of employment uncertainty at the end of a project. Everyone who worked on the project commented at their exit interview that they would miss the people – we enjoyed an incredible team spirit which built an enviable work culture. We accepted people from many countries whose backgrounds were different; yet we were all employed to abide by a set of common values, highlighting each person's self-acceptance of the project vision and behavioural compliance.

As the project finished the various stages in the Brisbane office, my role came to an end, and I decided to take an extended break as my adrenals were extremely low. I found it challenging to unwind. Five years of project life had kept me super busy, so relaxing to a slower pace was incredibly tricky. Acceptance of my current situation was difficult as I was usually up at 5 am and at work by 6.45 am, and now I had time to unwind, yet my thoughts kept wandering to the commissioning stage. A good friend suggested that on early rising that I go back to bed with a good book. I followed this advice when I awoke which allowed my mind to be absorbed in the respective book's places and events and she was right – it worked, and slowly I accepted the changes to my daily life. I felt that I needed some stimulation while unwinding and decided that a life coaching qualification would be a great skill set to accompany my HR experience. I enrolled in an Advanced Practitioner in Life Coaching with a provider based in Melbourne. Before the course commenced, other things occurred during that year which I couldn't initially understand or comprehend, as it felt like I was in a long dark tunnel. Thomas Moore describes it as a black sea where we see the vast potential of life, but it was my dark night.[27] I took the 'dark night of my soul' description literally and wondered why it continued for the best part of several months and not one night. My project position had contributed to a healthy ego which unravelled to bring me back to my primordial self, my original self: seeing myself as a sea of possibility, my higher and deeper self. This phase of my life brought much change and transformational moments intertwined with learning, fun and pleasure as the dark stage lifted.

Four one-week coaching intensives took me to Melbourne regularly during that year, and I met some fantastic people who were also on the coaching program. Many of these friendships continue, and the support given to us by the tutors was lovely, as they provided excellent feedback on our coaching techniques. Awareness opened for continual personal growth and knowledge as I trained to be a life coach, as I had to observe and accept myself in each program segment. My colleagues were terrific, as they understood that at times I was going through another process, and their support and coaching helped me navigate through the ups and downs of this particular journey. There were times when I despaired; tears flooded my face. I questioned my self-worth. My fluctuating emotions saw my mind grappling with why I had made these choices. Some days were a real struggle to get out of bed; I just wanted to turn over and forget the issues which played on my mind.

Looking back, this became a year of incremental change; albeit including times of very low moments. During the coaching program, I started my own business to provide HR and coaching services. All of this was a new experience and was very grounding and humbling to look at all the different hats I would wear to make my business viable. It took lots of research about ASIC (Australian Securities and Investments Commission), to register a company with a name not already in use. This became a year to learn all about how to launch a small business.

---

27 Thomas Moore, 2004, *Dark Nights of the Soul*, p5

At this stage, I dug deep into my inner journey to face the dark night of the soul process which probed every aspect of my being, bringing pain as well as deliverance. It was a very personal journey facing a *'long series of locks that lift us up to take us down to a new plateau'.*[28] During this time of soul refinement, I shed many tears in my inner search to acknowledge a deepening of intelligence. Moore explains the clear difference between considering depression as being a mood and a dark night is a process. Carl E Rogers has a quote which I find describes it perfectly: *'The curious paradox is that when I accept myself just as I am, then I can change.'*

Change within myself was endless... patterns fell away as I explored new options to grow within myself. It was allowing what is not working, serving or supporting me, to drop, that provided an embrace of the new. There is no time like now to examine where you are and honestly feel into what is occurring. Life's rhythm doesn't play the same tune. Yes, we have our favourites until something new comes along, and we like that better. Same goes for living each moment of life.

Treasure nature and what it is telling us. Listen within to your intuition and take time to nurture yourself. It happens little by little, with small tasks repeated and having an open heart to make the change. Remove the veil from your eyes and look again at opportunities and what awaits in a new direction. Not everyone embraces change, yet those that do will reap the internal benefit and so too will those with whom they interact. Courage is required to want more and to heal oneself to grow. Similarly, I could compare my pattern to 'The Hero's Journey' outlined by Joseph Campbell: departure, initiation and return.

Becoming a Life Coach enhanced my intuitive skills as well as provided structure and new learnings. On reflection, education of the heart and mind assisted my soul's passage. Part of this journey

---

28 Thomas Moore, *Dark Nights of the Soul*, 2004, p23

shifted my attitude to death as a part of life I had known closed; through a vision I observed myself in a tower looking down at the lifeless me below; I was finding renewal in that dark night process. *"Care of the soul is not a surface activity; nor is it easy."*[29] I persisted with self-nurture and embraced changes to my health, work and play. I learned to love with my whole heart, without attachment to outcomes – through repetition, this enabled my soul to be strengthened.

Amongst all of this personal change, the world experienced the Global Financial Crisis (GFC). Employment was challenging in many areas, and people witnessed their investments and superannuation accounts sliced in half. Financially things were tight for me, and I envisaged that coaching, together with my HR skills, would pave the way for consulting. I made arrangements with a psychologist friend living in Singapore that we would join our expertise and provide training and coaching initiatives in Singapore and Australia. After visiting her to work through the details, she proudly announced that she was marrying her wonderful man and moving to France. I was very happy for her, and yet saddened that our plans and mutual consultancy would not eventuate for us. I accepted this change of events as no doubt this was not the path meant for me.

I verbalised the adage that when one door closes, another opens. I facilitated Happiness Seminars with a focus on positive psychology. I found deep rewards in preparation and delivery of these sessions and received great feedback on the content and activities. Together with some consultancy HR work on the Sunshine Coast and membership of the local Chamber of Commerce, Businesswomen's Networking Group and another business group, I was meeting lovely people in new environments. In all of these groups, it was imperative to get up and speak about one's business and have clear goals for outcomes. All of these steps were gradual and incremental, enabling immersion into new places with new people. Not necessarily transformational in the big scheme of things; yet it

29 Thomas Moore, *Dark Nights of the Soul*, 2004, p287

set the platform for acceptance of more profound inner work and believing in myself that I could do it!

Self-doubt about getting work became intense. I chased all sorts of leads with a lot of effort yet no traction. Some offerings were not quite the right fit for me. With engagement through my own company, I found small parcels of contracted work on the Sunshine Coast. During one business opportunity, I completed a business plan for a particular company which required some research into resource industry jobs. During this research, I found positions which aligned with my qualifications and experience, piquing my interest in full-time employment, especially after such lean times. Soon after I relocated to Townsville with a fly in/fly out HR Business Partner role, and it was exciting to be with a large organisation implementing massive change management, along with embedding a global cultural change to the business. I met many talented people in my professional capacity.

I didn't know anyone in Townsville and two lovely local ladies welcomed and accepted me into their life. To join in their family activities was super special. If you have ever relocated to another town, state or country, you will understand that finding friends and being accepted makes a world of difference with the transition. Townsville provided exploration and time to try new things like Yoga – which my body fails to sculpture – walking The Strand and Castle Hill, and doing Zumba classes. I attended renowned Dance North contemporary performance and felt exhilarated by their unique brand of dance inventiveness. I felt very blessed with the people who came into my life and the continuing caring and sharing of these friendships.

Before relocation to Townsville, I had signed up for a residential personal development course in the Maldives. Luckily for me, my new employer gave me leave to attend the pre-booked class. Set in a very nurturing yin (feminine) environment, I spent two weeks with people from around the world absorbing the course lectures, as well as a lot of time alone implementing the tools and doing the inner work. I have learned, *"Be considerate to yourself and put yourself first always; then you will do the same for others."*[30]

Many people question that comment when I share, often with an eyebrow raised and uncertain body language. I use the analogy of the safety video played on an airline: in the unlikely event that oxygen is required, oxygen masks will fall from the ceiling. Ensure you put on your own mask first before assisting anyone else. This is precisely the same thing. Help yourself first and when you feel able, help others. It is so important for me as I know that when I'm in a good place – emotionally, mentally, physically and spiritually – then whoever interacts with me will benefit. This interaction is across the board – family, business professionals and friends. As women, we often have that steady nurturing connection, and it takes discipline to realise that if we are not up to assisting others, *it is okay to say no.*

For a very long time, I felt an obligation to support and help others. Probably due to my belief system from childhood, I frequently put other's requirements before my own. I often helped others, even to my detriment – so strong was the mindset that my help was required. Maybe I thought that I needed to help, or 'rescue', that person. It reverted to me – how I was feeling about it and not necessarily whether the person wanted my assistance. Maybe it was emotionally about wanting to feel needed and accepted? Understand the difference between when it is okay to personally provide help and when it is okay to let support happen. Become aware of your self-care requirements. Set some time aside as this was a biggie for me to really understand my conditioning in my formative years and how that impacted on understanding it was okay to have time out for myself. Honour you – believe in your knowing.

During the Maldives residential inner work, I took the time to delve into my heart and action the teachings. It was during one of

---

30 Annette Noontil, *The Body is the Barometer of the Soul*, 2004, p33.

the dyad sessions that I became aware of being 'gullible'. My dyad partner was excellent and if I felt stuck, she would pose a question and get me back into the emotion. It was such a fantastic experience to actually *feel* the emotions that arose from the word and associated experiences and sit with it. Allowing the feelings to bubble up and to feel the anger, the knots in my stomach, the frustration, being inadequate, the sadness, being overly trusting, until there was nothing left to feel about 'gullible'. Something changes at that moment. After the process, a word flashed into my mind which gave me comfort. Truth. Truth as in if I am honest with myself, the truth will set me free.

In my situation, I was gullible to different stories which at the time caused my gut to question, which I ignored. Truth was my freedom; to believe in me, myself and my gut instinct. There was a lightness and a feeling of freedom. I celebrated this freedom by splashing in the beautiful Ari Atoll waters. Kuramathi Island nurtured my soul, and I transformed myself in many ways with like-minded people supporting each other in our journey. Process exercises were accomplished in isolation on the beach, with many dips in the aqua waters to refresh. On several occasions, small sharks swam past with bright, colourful fish. I felt safe and liberated. It was a time of deep reflection and growth – a gift to myself – which in turn gives me tools to empathise and support family, friends and clients. I experienced such gratitude on so many levels.

I share with you the procedure of "feeling" which made all the difference to how I process.

Take a situation which may be concerning you, let's say: feeling unworthy. Sit alone in a quiet spot in nature, perhaps the beach or on your balcony. Feel into the emotions that arise. It is essential to get out of your head (thoughts) and get into your heart (feeling) and just let the emotions arise. Feelings could be anger, frustration, I'm not important/ valued, belittled – whatever feelings occur, allow them to surface. It is one hundred percent important to sit with these feelings and let them arise – you may cry, you may scream, or you may laugh, or you may just feel raw. Let it all come out... it can take time, so please remove all time limits. When I first started this process, it would take me many hours. I kept getting into my head and not staying with the feeling. Acceptance of the situation is essential. Accept that you did the best you could do in the situation or condition or job or position that you are working through – do not judge yourself, just accept and let the feelings flow. Repeat this process until something changes within you. There is a shift that comes... sometimes a word comes to me, or a calm feeling. There is no right or wrong on how this will change – except that the feeling will change. Keep doing the process until there is nothing left to feel. You will know when you have success as I have found that the issue or feeling in question does not affect you anymore. Remember, if the pain or issue or problem has been with you for a long time, it may take longer process time to feel the shift over several sessions.

My self-development journey continued with a two-month on-line course, 'The Silent Revolution', by Jo Le Rose. Aspects of the course took us through step by step processes to understand the words we use, specifically the 'I, Me, My, and Mine' and the context in which we use them and the intent behind it. Something so simple can reveal so much. We then moved onto 'Sitting with Consciousness: Use the hand, body and mind exercise to grasp that you are not residing in these, only using them and perceive what's left. This is where you are residing, and your mind and body is a tool to be used by this great space of silence. Get used to sitting with it and being with it. If thoughts come into you as though from outside of your mind, i.e. something you haven't thought up yourself, then this is consciousness using the mind! Pay attention.'[31] The course looked deeply into oneself to facilitate self-acceptance as well as achievement on set tasks. The tasks were varied, challenging and exciting.

---

31 Jo Le Rose, *The Silent Revolution*, Worksheet and University of Consciousness Education Certificate in Client Transformation https://uceducation.online/

On the final webinar, Jo conducted a visualisation, and it remains one of the most transformational moments of my life. The culmination of the self-work manifested for me in a fantastic realisation that I connected to my higher self. During the guided meditation by Jo, my Internet connection waned and I lost the sound. I called a girlfriend who placed her phone near her laptop so that I could hear the words and follow the visualisation. At the end of Jo's dialogue, I felt myself figuratively stretching higher and higher and then I connected with my spiritual guides – my father and soon after, my paternal and maternal grandmothers appeared. It was a moment of pure euphoria! I've known for some time that my father has been with me as a spiritual guide, and if I wake early in the morning, I can chat to him. It was a surprise to see my grandmothers – such a special moment and one that I will cherish. Something changed within me during that process. It is hard to find words that convey the deep connection and love that occurred in that process. My energy vibrated at a different frequency, and I experienced heights of joy and elation beyond description. I soared in this space for about three weeks as the transformation was sublime and empowering. I still smile recalling this event which is indelibly etched in my memory. As described by Cassandra Sturdy: *'Your "vibration" is a fancy way of expressing your overall state of being. Everything in the universe is made up of energy vibrating at different frequencies. Even things that look solid are made up of vibrational energy fields at the quantum level. This includes you.'*[32]

We have different energy levels: physical, mental, emotional and spiritual. From a scientific and metaphysical perspective, these levels have a vibrational frequency which align to our state of wellbeing. Sometimes our frequency is low as perhaps we are not taking care of ourselves, or something outside of our control has impacted us intellectually, and our response is not one of love. During this period of connection with my higher self, I soared at a

---

32 https://www.theholisticingredient.com/blogs/wholesome-living/13587702-8-ways-to-raise-your-vibration-your-positive-energy

high vibration as I was in the true flow of life. Through my positive approach to life and in establishing healthy and kind habits, I live a life that is fulfilling. Of course, I have rare times when I may want to have a 'pity party', yet no one wants to be part of that process – not even me – and I quickly change the lens that I look through to one of optimism and love. It takes a fraction of time to change my outlook. The results are astounding.

I am aware that what brings us joy raises our vibration. My love of dancing gives me immense pleasure, and my energy levels increase as my endorphins are popping to the bopping! What do you do that brings you joy? Be in that joy with certainty and in that energy of who you are now. If you are not feeling in alignment and your joy is diminished, it might be helpful to recognise the situation (you can add names, places and more details) and choose to release the outcome. You can release the issue to the universe, your god or to whomever you place your faith. Offer thanks for this guidance. Be sure of the outcome and leave your anxiety behind. I sometimes use the phrase – let go and let God. What is the phrase that will serve you best?

Another way to feel worthy and gain acceptance is to offer appreciation. Abraham Hicks' Technique is the Appreciation Game, and Gabby Bernstein recommends it as well. Words and action spread appreciation, and it clears the past.

The game is simple yet powerful:

1. Tell someone what you appreciate about them.

2. Then they tell you.

3. You tell them something else.

4. Keep it up for a minute or two.

This technique lifts both people very quickly, raising vibration and has been proven to dissolve tension and lead to resolution faster.

During 2017 another change occurred as I woke during a dream. It is unusual for me to recall my dreams, and this time it was in full technicolour, and it appeared as two people joined as one. My first thought was that a man would enter my life. That was a momentary assumption as one half lifted their head and I saw long blond hair. The face did not have detail, yet on closer introspection I realised that it was me – I felt that it represented the male and female aspects of me joined. I was complete and balanced with my male and feminine energy. For a long time, the masculine energy was dominant in my life. Being a workaholic made this the prevailing aspect. My feminine side has always been within me and perhaps not as dominant as the male energy. Since that dream, I know that I am enough for myself – I am complete. These words may seem harsh – it does not mean that I do not need anyone in my life; it tells me that I have everything that I require within my being. I have self-acceptance.

Action Aces

▶ Have there been times in your life when you felt unworthy?

▶ What emotions did the feelings raise?

▶ Follow the exercise summary for feeling 'unworthy.'

  • *Sit alone in a quiet spot in nature*

  • *Allow the emotional feelings to come from your heart If your mind comes into play, remove the thoughts and concentrate on the feelings*

  • *Feelings could be anger, frustration, feeling belittled or disappointed*

  • *Sit with the emotions and let them genuinely expand so that you are really in the energy*

  • *Do not judge yourself – just feel and accept this was what happened*

  • *Keep feeling the emotions until something changes Repeat the process until there is no unworthy emotion to rise*

▶ Raising your vibration – to keep your vibration high, maintain unconditional love and look for the good in all situations. Play the Appreciation Game and see if it raises your vibration.

▶ Clear the subconscious with 11 x 22s exercise – eleven consecutive days with positive 'I' sentences to release distorted energy. Write sentence twenty-two times with whatever thought pops into your mind after the positive start. Do not re-read your sentences. Discard the written words daily.

For example:

1. I am perfectly acceptable as I am *even when I doubt myself.*
2. I am perfectly acceptable as I am *in each moment.*

Another Sentence for Acceptance: **I am equal to all life...**

Clearing Your Subconscious 11 x 22's:

- *The subconscious is stored within our cells.*
- *The process of using numbers with repeated affirmative sentences can break down a belief pattern.*
- *On an energetic level, the positive words enter into the mind and body, pushing out distorted energy.*
- *An internal shift then occurs as the distortion is dispersed through the aura, leaving it clear.*

CHAPTER FIVE

Feeling Self Doubt – Gaining Confidence

"Reach within to find your strength and the task becomes easy."

Anne Poole

Have you heard the phrase 'fake it until you make it'? What feelings arise within you when you read that?

That phrase intends to raise your confidence level to remove self-doubt. Sounds easy – right? For some of us, it is a lot harder to achieve. Self-doubt prevents us from reaching our full potential. Self-doubt leaves us struggling to believe in our own strengths. When we are in that mindset, we strive to feel good internally, and externally it is displayed in how we present ourselves. Did you know that when we meet someone, it takes about 6 seconds to form an opinion about that person? It is our subconscious kicking into action. For example, if you met a hiring manager for a job interview, you have 6 seconds to make an impression before opening your mouth – how would you prepare? Would you consider things like – washed hair, clean fresh face, wide smile, eye to eye contact, tidy appearance – wearing shoes rather than thongs (flip flops)? How you prepare through hygiene and presentation will also give you a confidence boost. Try it and see how you feel if you do these things. Simple, yet how you feel makes the difference. The hiring manager perceives you through the care you have taken in your appearance. That could translate into how you might present at work and do your tasks—considering that self-care also makes the shift within your mind.

I have found that when my hair is washed and clean, I feel confident. Such a little thing to do for myself, yet it has a huge impact. Some ladies might find if they have applied makeup, that enhances their confidence. Find whatever it is that gives you a boost and ensure you make it part of your routine. It makes a noticeable difference in how you feel inside. Gaining confidence usually takes time, although some people appear to have buckets of confidence. Some are very blessed with talented genes, some are maybe faking it until they make it, others have put in a lot of work to be competent in a chosen field, which gives them confidence.

When we judge others, compare ourselves to others, and attack others, we see ourselves as separate. Sometimes with our feelings of self-doubt, we go into the blame game and start comparisons with others. When you are in that state – *stop*, and take care of you. Gaining confidence is a time to be gentle, as well as honest.

Allow me to share a particular occasion when I worked for a public utility company where I was employed as a Human Resources (HR) consultant using my recruitment skills and broad HR knowledge to bring a project to fruition. Each member of the team had a full workload plus a myriad of team building activities that were implemented to bind this new team together. The delegation gave me some big tasks which I took in my stride and felt I was delivering, yet it became clear to me and others, that I was being singled out a little at work. We had an open-plan office with about eight to ten of us in the space. The manager was able to view each member of her team. Sometimes we chatted about status and other times we fielded responses via emails. In front of everyone, I was asked: 'What's the status of the preferred supplier's list for recruiters?' Then, in a demanding tone, 'What's happening with the sample uniform selection process?' I felt intimidated being put on the spot in front of the whole team. The manager's tone and behaviour towards me in front of the group impacted me greatly. A couple of other team members looked at me with empathy, as well as relief that it wasn't them being targeted.

As the manager's scrutiny towards each project portfolio I was handling intensified, a part of my confidence unravelled each day. I dreaded going to work. Usually, I would bounce out of bed and couldn't wait for the day to start and had already planned my 'to do' list. Now my emotions were electrified – and more like a slow, creeping burn feeling than a high energy. I thought that I was not good enough, not giving enough, and it did impact my performance. My self-doubt was in full swing. Have you ever felt this way? I spiralled to feeling as though I was an incompetent worker. Normally I am a high achiever, and I couldn't understand why I was receiving phone calls from this manager at 9.45 pm at night, asking about a recruitment strategy recommendation. I usually wouldn't answer the phone at that hour, so I thought it must be an emergency. There were other phone calls at night and one in particular occurred during a Friday evening event, with her demanding to know why I was not in attendance. It was communicated that I was letting the team down, and yet only one other HR team member attended. I responded that while it was an optional attendance work event, my friends were arriving via train for the weekend and I was collecting them. On reflection, I could have sent my apologies due to previous commitments, yet in my anxious state that had not occurred to me. In hindsight, I feel this was the turning point as the manager felt deserted by the team, and I was the unfortunate person on the receiving end of her wrath.

According to the Australian Human Rights Commission, the situation in which I found myself has a label – 'workplace bullying'. The legislative definition is 'The repeated less favourable treatment of a person by another or others in the workplace, which may be considered unreasonable and inappropriate workplace practice.' I endured this behaviour without speaking up. Fear gripped me and my self-doubt intensified. In my mind, I concluded that because my Manager and the CEO were close that I might not have a fair hearing. Generally, in a workplace situation, if you cannot speak to your manager, (or your manager is the problem) you go to Human Resources. We were Human Resources. Protocols typically come into effect, and it goes to the next organisational level, which in this instance would have been the CEO. I will never know how that might have played out, as I was called to a meeting to talk about my performance or supposed lack thereof. I felt it better to simply leave and I resigned during that meeting. I felt humiliated and alone.

Of course, this experience impacted my confidence immensely, and it also left me with a feeling that within the workplace I was not competent. I felt singled out and subjected to ridicule, persistent and unjustified criticisms, and intimidation via the evening phone calls. From my HR experience, I have investigated workplace bullying situations, and it is not pleasant for anyone. In mature organisations, there is a process which is clearly outlined to all staff on employment commencement and which provides the mechanism to chat about perceived behaviours. Now, I have finally spoken up. While it is never easy to find the courage to speak to HR or a senior person about the issue, speaking up is the highest priority. In the space of ten years since this occurred, our Australian communities are far more aware of what workplace bullying entails and what constitutes unacceptable behaviour.

I also know that the 'fast writing' technique would have been a benefit to me during and after my work situation – just writing down all the anger, frustration and hurt that the job gave me. It is essential to know that fast writing is a great mechanism to give voice to the thoughts inside our head. The process is named fast writing, as you just keep expressing your emotional feelings onto paper. Never read over what you have written – it only brings it up again – instead just burn it or dispose through soaking in water and placing the paper in an outside rubbish bin. Speaking to a trusted friend also can assist in sharing the burden. Sometimes coaching is required as the effects of bullying can hide deep within us, and we need to release this and find the root cause with a skilled professional.

My healing process involved visualisations and meditation and doing the 11 x 22s. See **Action Aces** for details. Another tool for dissipating anger is to go outside in a wide-open space. Standing with feet slightly apart, place your hands into a fist in front of the heart and press tightly together. Locking your hands together allows for you to tense your clenched fists. As you start breathing fast – breathe in and breathe out quickly as you keep thinking of what made you angry or the emotional feelings within you. As you are doing this, tense your arms and shoulders so that your body is *feeling* the anger. Keep tensing until you can release it in front of you with a loud 'YAH!' and let go! Throw your hands out in front of you and let everything out. Repeat this process three times at a minimum. You can repeat in multiples of three – such as six or nine or twelve until it feels released. It may bring up some memories and you may also feel lightheaded.

My son said that he was not feeling well, and asked, could he stay home. Naturally, I thought he needed a day to recover if he had stomach pains. The next day he said he still had stomach pains. He was out of sorts and as a mother I knew that something wasn't right. I visited the school about his change of behaviour and asked could they observe him to find out if there was something at school which impacted his personality change. I also noticed that his love of martial arts had faded, and he was no longer keen to attend this extracurricular activity. The teachers at the school were caring. While I felt that twinge of self-doubt in my summation and maybe I was biased about my son, the teacher duly said she would observe what was occurring and come back to me. Within one week, teachers had identified situations occurring during lunch breaks. Once detected, we realised why there was no interest in the extracurricular activity. Thankfully, the situation resolved itself, and counselling took place. It pays to follow your self-doubt niggles, as there is value in what your gut is telling you.

Self-doubt occurred precisely on my fiftieth birthday: my car broke down at a bustling intersection. It was confronting. Hello universe – I am being given a situation. To me, my car is an analogy of my life journey. Every time I got into my car; my thoughts went to *'What if I break down?'* Mechanics tested my car and found no real issues and still it just conked out at any time, at any place. I began to dread driving. I left the vehicle with the mechanic for three weeks while I travelled overseas. On my return, the mechanic said only once did my car just stop for an unknown reason. I felt vindicated! I also thought it was time to replace that car.

What this scenario highlighted to me is that what we focus on, we get! I was concentrating on my car, breaking down, and sure enough, it did. Émile Coué, the French psychologist and mind theorist, devised a simple mantra-based method to reprogram your psyche along the lines of confidence, wellness and enthusiasm. I have used this affirmation to change my life as the positive words relate to every aspect of living. For example, from a straightforward thing like my Latin dancing: 'I now have more confidence when dancing with partners and instructors during lessons.' The mantra is the only thing that I can attribute the change to – other than attending weekly lessons. His work predates the works of Anthony Robbins as well as clinical developments in neuro, sleep, placebo and psychical research. You may have heard this mantra, yet not be aware it came from Coué, who was also a hypnotherapist and psychologist:

'Day by day, in every way,
I am getting better and better.'[33]

---

33 Émile Coué, 2019, *Self Mastery Through Conscious Autosuggestion*, p30

Our thoughts flow onto feelings, and I have become incredibly aware of the power of our mind. It is crucial to be clear on our focus. Understand the intent behind it. Is it pure? I share an example which might provide clearness. Many years ago, I believed that if I did a good turn for someone, then I would expect that it would be reciprocated when I needed it. It is a belief that was culturally strong and somewhere I had picked up that if you go the extra mile for someone, well, they will go the extra mile for you when required. No, no, no. When I go the extra mile for someone now, it is on my terms. I want to serve or assist that person with no strings attached. Even if they do not say thank you, it is okay because I gave of my time and/or talents willingly to assist that person and I was not attached to any outcome – be it financial payment, reciprocal gift or whatever. Do you understand? I render help irrespective of the result. To me, the above explains 'not attached to an outcome'. Once I became aware of what I was doing, there was a shift in my focus and my confidence to offer unconditional gifts. However, it is not to say that I give everything away – I invoice for my services – yet there are times when I want to freely give.

When I was a Girl Guide, I was given ten laws to learn, and it was a guideline on how to live your best life as a Guide. The tenth law was: *'A Guide is pure in thought, word and deed.'* My realisation of this law came to me immediately when I discovered about giving and not seeking a return. It honestly took on profound transparency. As a teenager, it was easy to repeat the laws by rote, yet as an adult, each word was not just memorisation; it held meaningful wisdom.

Take the time now to think about: what you do for others and is there is an expectation of a reward or a return favour?

Accept yourself in this response. If you thought that because you were friendly and gave so much time to assist that person, was it okay to believe that they would repay you for your kindness? Many of us have followed family beliefs or traditions from our ancestors without ever questioning why we do it. What is your belief? How will you approach your acts of kindness in the future? Listen to your intuition.

I became aware that my inner voice – inner wisdom, gut feeling, or intuition – was guiding me. I believe that our inner voice does not know right and wrong – it just knows. I am convinced that our inner voice or feeling is like a compass showing us the path or direction. I have observed that if I follow that feeling, all aspects work out. Getting in touch with this inner voice is getting to know yourself – spending time in nature, focussing on the breath, slowing down to be in each moment – allows for us to listen to these feelings. I wanted to develop this intuition muscle, and I've tried it in all sorts of situations. Many times, I have called on my inner voice to assist me in finding a car park. Yes, an everyday occurrence: it has led me to a car park that is close to the entrance or to a vacant parking spot that I didn't even know existed – I trusted my inner voice. Of course, if there is not a park, I am directed to go to another area; I follow. This example highlights a simple way to build the muscle of trusting one's inner voice; not to mention finding a parking spot quickly.

I used this inner voice as I explored London during my fiftieth year and revisited places I'd seen some thirty years previously. I also found the courage to find and attend St Martin in the Fields at Trafalgar Square to listen to beautiful classical music. I believed that I would attend. Success – venue located and my confidence was high. There was a time when I couldn't read a map – I turned it upside down to get clear about which direction. Many refer to this as a female trait: yet I was quite determined to find this venue by myself and follow the map. I enjoyed such a memorable performance within this lovely church. For some, doing these things is like riding a bike – just get back on and go – yet for me, at times doing the unknown can bring an unsettled, transient feeling. I have also learned that to take a deep breath calms me very quickly as I focus only on the breath, and then I feel confident to follow my inner voice. You might like to try what has worked for me: take three deep breaths through the nose to the solar plexus and slowly release through the mouth. Experiment with this and work out what your body requires to feel the calmness that stilling the mind through breath-work can bring.

For a long time, I had been searching for a place on the Sunshine Coast – possibly Caloundra as it held special childhood memories of times with my parents at Golden Beach and Bulcock Beach. One particular morning, I found a small advert for a private sale for a unit four hundred metres from the beach. My heart pumped, yet I could not make the viewing that morning – I didn't have a vehicle. I phoned the number from the advert, and the gentleman said he would meet me the following Saturday. I secured a lift with a friend, and on arrival just felt that the energy of the unit was perfect. I loved the ocean views, the rooftop provided space for growing herbs and fruit trees in pots, my washing could dry in the sun and breeze – it had forty-five stairs – yes, that's manageable, and it would keep me fit as I aged. My friend insisted that I look at other properties. Self-doubt rose within me as I truly felt that this was '*the* unit'. My friend showed kindness and business savvy by insisting on viewing other properties. I mulled over the advantages and disadvantages of each place. While self-doubt initially prevailed, a more energetic feeling within me led to my decision to make an offer on the original unit. I firmly believe that when all the doors open, then it is meant to be. I give gratitude for my decision and confidence to purchase. I am truly blessed as I write my book from this beautiful home.

I have found that creativity boosts my confidence. All of us have a creative streak – it shows in how we approach many aspects of our life. Some exhibit creativity through the arts – painting, cake icing, singing, decorating, designing gardens, furniture, or fabrics, others through problem-solving – finding solutions, innovative leadership and imagination for film and music. Creativity exists in many aspects of my life, and I enjoy the challenge of solving problems with lateral thinking, as well as taking courses to quench my thirst for knowledge.

Still in my fiftieth celebration year, I explored my creativity and attended a painting class in France with my talented friend Sophia Flowers. During this creative sanctuary, I naturally detoxed: I had a full-blown cold, and my lungs removed lots of unwanted gunk. In the art class, I found myself feeling very structured, and it took almost the entire week's course for me to unwind and allow myself to 'let go', and I produced my own style of Monet's garden. I found that my creativity was stilted. I was caged and kept myself invisible. Taking a painting class was way out of my comfort zone. A good friend told me recently that 'You certainly like a challenge, Anne!' I hadn't quite appreciated that was how I came across, yet when I thought about it, it was true. The painting class was a demonstration of my wanting to 'get it right' and yet my imagination was narrow and stilted when putting colours onto paper in an eye-pleasing manner. It didn't matter what kind of artwork I produced on each of the five days – I explored a part of me that was full of self-doubt, and it showed through each of the five paintings. Each day I could see the progression as I found confidence and freedom in doing whatever felt appropriate for the subject matter. Without a doubt, I gained confidence each day in an unknown medium and environment.

I had visited Monet's Garden just before coming to the course as I stayed with my daughter-in-law's parents in Orly, Paris. The gardens inspired me on so many levels, with the colour, natural flow of plants – edible as well as purpose-planted for riots of colour. The bees were in heaven with the floral abundance, and I too was thrilled to visit the home of one my favourite artists. It was breathtaking; despite my high expectations, I wasn't disappointed. With a bilingual guide, I enjoyed asking many questions about Monet and his residence, including his art collection beside the gardens. A cultural feast of design and flora. Très bon!

During my stay in the Pays de la Loire region of France, I walked alongside beautiful tall trees and babbling brooks and enjoyed being a tourist. During the Bob Ross Art tutorials, my eyes feasted on rolling hills and open spaces, magnificent sunrises and engagement with Tai Chi and Chi Gong morning exercises. Each experience taught me more about myself and the journey of self-discovery and acceptance through exploring creativity with paint on canvas. I was well and truly out of my comfort zone – and that was a good thing as the painting class allowed me to express where I was at that moment in time, and I could appreciate what it was showing me.

Conversely, I'm in my comfort zone when I do HR processes. I love to introduce effective and efficient ways to tackle a topic and streamline implementation with Lean Principles (associated with Six Sigma). I love the facilitation process with a small group to brainstorm a problem and then funnelling the ideas into tangible options. The creativity from each person brings a richness of views and expanse of thoughts from varied experience and cultures, which give confidence for others to join in the discussions.

On many occasions, I have enjoyed making quilts and other various items doing patchwork – assembling colours and shapes to perfection (or non-perfection!) to dazzle the eye and provide either stimulation or reflective moments. Patchwork is like art with putting colours together, yet there are patterns available to follow for designs leaving the colour placement my own choice. I designed some of my clothes using patchwork techniques, and that was lots of fun. I was happy with my creations, and my self-confidence increased when I received compliments.

A long time ago, I saw corkboards displayed in a magazine – it stimulated my imagination as it was using wine and champagne corks. I hadn't realised how many corks would be required just for one corkboard. Friends rallied around and kept drinking wine and champers to build my cork collection! Wow, did I receive. Much gratitude to my friends. Thank goodness they indulged, as wine corks disappeared with the introduction of screw tops. I also assembled cork boards utilising the wine and champagne corks onto beautiful bespoke timber frames from my woodturners, Frank and Clare. I enjoyed lots of creativity sessions, as well as completing gifts for special people in my life.

Creativity removes blockages, allows problem-solving to occur, and if I go within myself, I find insights and answers. Everyone will have an opinion: it is not good nor bad, it just is. Trusting in your abilities will strengthen your muscle by following your intuition or inner guidance. Creativity occurs in so many areas of our life – preparing a meal, decorating a home, thinking outside the square, dance, movement, gardening, and the list goes on.

- What area of creativity captures your interest?

- How do you feel it enriches your life?

- List some ideas for an experiment.

A fresh burst of energy and confidence entered my life during my fifties. As women, we go through hormonal changes, and while I never exhibited any external signs of menopause, my doctor monitored my progress through blood tests. One of the many learnings about this stage of my life was reframing the opportunity to look at menopause. Essentially, it is a time of rebirth. It was such an opportunity to monitor the changes as I embraced each step anew. It certainly let me go deeper within to explore and understand many of the childhood issues and see it as an opportunity to bring change, healing and closure. It was a time to feel renewed as I journeyed this stage in my life. I found it uplifting to know that I had another chance at life and as so much occurred in my fiftieth year, this focus on rebirth allowed a different approach. My focus had changed, which put a confident spring in my step.

With the modern advances in technology, it is possible to do many courses online and have global group discussions easily, quickly and economically. I joined Chi Gong, and each week there is a new online video for exercises. These gentle exercises focus on creating calmness within one's life, breathing, and touches on mindfulness and the benefits that it brings. Whether it is Yoga or Chi Gong or another modality that brings you back to concentration on the breath, it all aids in living in harmony with nature and grounding us to feel a calm confidence within ourselves.

I trust that my memoirs will be thought-provoking. While your situation may be different from mine, our journeys may be similar in scenarios and mindsets, which impact gaining confidence. Below are tools to help you in your journey through the **Action Aces** and always, the answers are within!

Action Aces

- ▶ Have you noticed when you feel confident in your appearance? What did you do to make you feel that way?

- ▶ Conversely, are you aware of when your appearance affects your confidence?

- ▶ What small step can you take to improve your confidence?

- ▶ Fast writing – release your emotional feelings through fast writing. Do not re-read; just dispose of safely.

- ▶ Émile Coué's mantra: *'Day by day, in every way, I am getting better and better.'* Each morning on waking and each evening before sleep, repeat mantra twenty times.

- ▶ Clear the subconscious with 11 x 22s exercise – eleven consecutive days with positive 'I' sentences to release distorted energy. Write sentence twenty-two times with whatever thought pops into your mind after the positive start. Do not re-read your sentences. Discard the written words daily.

For example:

1. I am fulfilling my life purpose, and I have great joy and happiness *in each moment.*

2. I am fulfilling my life purpose, and I have great joy and happiness *when I'm feeling lost.*

Another Sentence for Confidence: **I am equal to all life...**

Clearing Your Subconscious 11 x 22s:

- *The subconscious is stored within our cells.*

- *The process of using numbers with repeated affirmative sentences can break down a belief pattern.*

- *On an energetic level, the positive words enter into the mind and body, pushing out distorted energy.*

- *An internal shift then occurs as the distortion is dispersed through the aura, leaving it clear.*

CHAPTER 6

Feeling Inner Voice – Gaining Intuition

INTUITION

Intuition connects us to self-trust, enabling us to embrace the unknown and act from the heart's recognition of truth rather than the mind's need for certainty.

Jilly Gabrielson, Bright Spark Health

Jilly expresses the word "IN TU I TION" as dissected to mean suggesting, delving inwards – an act of sensing beyond what is outwardly visible and palpable. (In to I [self] – ion is a doing). I love this!

"The intellect has little to do on the road to discovery. There comes a leap in consciousness, call it intuition or what you will, and the solution comes to you, and you don't know how or why."

Albert Einstein, Physicist

Your intuition is your internal compass... do you agree?

If you agree, you know that your intuition is your true north. It does not know "right" or "wrong". It only knows what is best for you.

Do you ask others for insight/advice into your life, career, and partner?

I've done that. Yet, when I take the time alone, I realise that all the answers are within.

When you trust your gut feeling, know you are on your best path.

In the earlier chapters, I spoke about intuition and provided examples of how it has been a great signal in my life. One of the exercises is to do a simple "yes" or "no" exercise. Getting clear on this is vital to building the intuitive muscle. The exercise is found at the end of this chapter's **Action Aces**.

Most of us will have a body response to our "gut feeling," "sixth sense," or "instinct."

Firstly, what is intuition? Intuition is often described as understanding or knowing something without conscious reasoning. It's a subconscious process that draws on patterns, experiences, and knowledge stored in our minds.

In the past, many shirked away from practising the art of intuition as it was considered mysterious and perhaps more for eccentrics. Attitudes have changed over the years. The rational mind is more considered the sphere of intellect and is given prominence, often called the masculine mind. Conversely, the feminine mind was considered intuitive. Intuition communicates as a hunch, a gut feeling, or an inner voice speaking to you. Intuition is non-linear. We do not receive rules or a program to follow.

This innate capability allows you to make decisions swiftly and effectively, especially when faced with ambiguity or incomplete information.

Your intuition is not a random feeling but a product of your accumulated expertise and situational awareness. It manifests as a gut feeling, a sudden insight, or a hunch that guides decision-making.

Importantly, it complements analytical thinking, providing immediate, instinctual responses that can be just as valid and valuable as a well-reasoned analysis.

By understanding the nature of intuition and its significant role in decision-making, you can tap into its power to enhance rational analysis.

This balanced approach can empower you to make more effective and efficient decisions, bolstering your confidence in your abilities.

Your inner voice may also prompt you. Something pops into your mind – for example, an outdoor screen near the spa. Mmmm, I'm not sure what that is about. It's a windy day, and you tell yourself, I'll bring the screen in later. Bang! The screen falls over. You didn't follow the prompts immediately, yet your intuition gave you signals! I'm sure you know how it works now, and you will listen to that inner voice as it is your intuition.

Early in my human resources career, I recall being aware that one of the chosen candidates for a senior management role didn't come across as ideal. He was liaising with me on various issues regarding his onboarding, housing, and overall package. My antenna was alerted. Something didn't feel quite right. My manager must have observed my reluctance to say too much and asked, "Do you think we have chosen the wrong candidate?" I told my manager that something was amiss. He asked why. I told him it was my intuition and gave him my rationale.

This manager came on board, and within two months, my observations were evident to the executive team. The usual process was applied, and he was made aware of his behaviours. No change occurred within the set timeframe, and he left.

Intuitive insights can facilitate understanding unspoken cues or underlying motivations in team dynamics or negotiations.

Intuition can spark creativity and unconventional ideas that data analysis alone might not uncover.

In scenarios where data is limited or ambiguous, intuition can fill in the gaps by drawing on past experiences and patterns.

While looking through Facebook, I recently read an article that impacted me. Sasha is an entrepreneur running her business on Queensland's Sunshine Coast. She runs a dance studio incorporating significant events, catering, fashion, and wellness. Her post reflected on the recent successful event. Sasha has kindly permitted me to share.

"A heart full of gratitude and also peace. But this is not the case in every event that I have done.

The last time I did an event in this venue was a very different story. After the massive showcase was done and everyone had cleared out of the green room, I was there alone and burst into tears. I ran the biggest event of my life with an audience of 500+. We ran a bar and my company also catered! The event was so busy, a bit chaotic but all in all a massive success and at the time I had no idea why I felt so empty and sad.

The biggest lessons I have learnt over the past couple of years in business and in my personal life is that intuition is everything. Most of the time your body knows before your mind catches up. Your body knows when something is not right, when you are not truly supported by the people working closely with you, when people smiling in your face and then being shit behind your back.

Cut to this year, not one ounce of sadness or my intuition screaming at me. I could not have asked for a better show, for better people surrounding me-audience, students and teachers. I feel blessed from the bottom of my soul to be able to have this experience, to have the opportunity and the support to make this contribution to the arts and represent Brazilian culture in the best way that I can."

Well done, Sasha, for your successful event and sharing your emotions. You listened to your body and intuition. You surrounded yourself with supportive people. You make an outstanding contribution to Brazilian culture through dance performances and lessons.

You can be like Sasha, tuning into your body signals and "knowing" your choices are perfect for you. Hollie Azzopardi writes in her book, The People Pleaser's Guide to Putting Yourself First, that *"your intuition will never "should" on you, ever!" p113*

You are a brilliant, intuitive person whose "inner compass" is designed to help you "know" things. Each of us was born with this skill. Today, more and more people are exploring it and not bowing down to the overly masculine energy of worshipping the pragmatic and logical. I'm not saying there is not a place for pragmatism and logic. There is. Over the years, our intuition has communicated softly, and there is not so much in the public mainstream environment.

How can you build your intuition?

- I have found time in nature is a great foundation. Walking in the bush, forest, and beach allows us to have reflective time to observe and listen.

- Keeping a journal can assist us. Writing down our feelings when our body niggles tell us about a "yes" or a "no" response. Become familiar with how your body lets you know will build your intuitive muscle.

- Start with an easy exercise, and ask your inner voice to help you find your phone, car keys, or glasses. Yes, it's an everyday occurrence, as we often misplace these. I've trusted myself and followed my gut; yes, there is my phone. Keep doing this, and believe your intuition will tell you where to find your misplaced object. This builds the muscle of trusting your inner voice and finding that vital object.

- Intuition often nudges towards growth areas where you can expand your skills and expertise.

- Look closely at the areas of work that consistently excite and engage you.

- Intuition often aligns with passion, indicating your natural strengths and interests.

- Meditation stills the mind, allowing for the mind's natural curiosity to be heard. Sometimes, it will be tranquil; other meditation times reveal awareness of situations. The more you quiet the mind, the better your intuition will give you signals.

There are pros and cons to intuition.

Advantages include:

- Facilitating quick decision-making,

- Fostering creativity and

- Sometimes gaining a competitive edge.

Disadvantages include:

- The possibility that reliance on intuition may pose risks due to biases, emotional influences, and

- Overconfidence may cloud judgment and potentially lead to suboptimal decisions.

Understanding the pros and cons of intuition promotes a holistic approach to decision-making that integrates intuitive insights with analytical rigour.

These pros and cons are almost non-existent as you build your intuitive muscle`. Initially, when I realised I was getting these "feelings", I wasn't sure what I was feeling and was a little sceptical about voicing my concern. With time, I now know that my intuitive niggles and feelings are spot on for my path.

In some interview processes, I have struggled with judging a person. I only have the resume, cover letter, emails, and the interview to decide. Sometimes, personality testing can be helpful, yet I only use it as one instrument in selecting candidates. Luckily, there is always an interview panel, which means robust discussions evolve and our concerns are discussed. Once you have secured that dream job, you may be confronted in the workplace with unfair judgement. This can be disheartening and challenging to navigate. It can stem from biases, misunderstandings, or subjective perceptions. Take a moment to recall when you felt that unfair judgement that impacted your morale and productivity. Many of us have experienced it. Your intuition can help you recognise subtle cues and underlying motivations and constructively guide responses.

Reflect on your feelings and reactions, as that is how intuition surfaces. Take time to identify how you feel about the situation and why. Often, self-awareness clarifies your perspective and guides your next step.

Intuitive insights can be validated by seeking feedback from trusted colleagues or mentors. You can hear their viewpoint and constructive criticism that assists you in understanding your situation.

Use your intuition to choose a thoughtful response. Take time to process what has occurred and tell the person. "I'll come back to you. I need to consider what you said." Maintaining professionalism is paramount, as once your words are spoken, they may have long-term implications.

Equally, there may be times when you have a hunch about a person or situation. For example, you may recall a lady who did not want to take a plane trip because she was experiencing nightmares before the trip. Friends and family said this is a trip of a lifetime, and these are your dreams. She was experiencing déjà vu. Sadly, that plane went down and has never been found. This story highlights that what your intuition tells you is for your best interests: no one else, just you. It is imperative to remember this.

Your intuition is your compass for direction. This is why I say the answers are within. Once you develop these inherent skills that have often lain dormant, you will know that these body signals are in your best interests for guidance.

Action Aces

▶ Take time in nature to observe and be still. Listen to the sounds around you, feel the breeze, smell the forest or bush or saltwater, look at the horizon or the abundance of flora and fauna. Close your eyes and focus on breathing in, breathing out, breathing in, breathing out, breathing in and breathing out. Repeat this regularly as it allows the sixth sense to develop.

▶ Start with an easy exercise: ask your inner voice to help you find your house keys. I've trusted myself and followed my gut; yes, there are my house keys. Keep doing this and believe that your intuition will find your misplaced object. This builds the muscle of trusting your inner voice and seeing that vital object.

▶ Write a journal about how you feel when you get negative vibes about something not for you. Similarly, write down the feelings that emerge when you have a positive "yes" to situations. Reflect on any patterns. Remember to date your journal to monitor the progress.

▶ Go outside or find a clear space inside the office or home. Use this exercise to help decipher what our intuition is saying to us. This is using your natural Chi. Stand with your legs slightly apart and ask the question with a "yes" or "no" response. An easy question is, "Is my name (insert what you are called)?" Because we have a natural chi energy field around us, you will notice that your chi energy moves somewhat forward or slightly backward. If your body sways forward, it acknowledges a "yes". If it pulls you slightly back, it answers "no".

▶ Do activities wherein your passion lies, and watch for the intuitive niggles that come from being in your place of bliss and fun.

CHAPTER SEVEN

Feeling Unheard – Finding Your Voice

"Try to say the very thing you really mean, the whole of it, nothing more or less or other than what you really mean. This is the whole art and joy of words."

C. S. Lewis

In life relationships, there have been times when I felt unheard. I would be involved in discussion with some friends and commence telling about an event, only to have my partner speak over me and finish what I had initiated. I felt my voice was taken away.

Did he not trust that I could finish the story?

Did he think that his version might be better than mine?

Did he feel that my voice was not required?

Have you been in that situation? Someone speaks over you before you have finished your sentence.

This behaviour has a controlling quality. In time, it spreads from just talking over you to controlling what you wear, or where you go and whom you are meeting. On the flip side, the person is unaware that they may even be doing it. Perhaps in the childhood family home, that behaviour was demonstrated. It is a modelled behaviour. If you feel into the emotion, it feels like a put-down. I felt not good enough. When it occurred repeatedly, it disturbed my equilibrium. I kept quiet and let the other person do the talking.

I do not recommend this approach for a healthy relationship. Communication is the key in any relationship – intimate or friendship or with work colleagues. Speaking to one another about what is occurring will often clarify the situation, and if identified early enough, there is a chance that it may foster change with more dialogue.

Earlier in the book, I mentioned my childhood conditioning and the belief that children should be seen and not heard and how it impacted my life. Finding my voice has included moments when I have taken charge and spoken out quickly and powerfully and other times when I have hidden my voice to avoid conflict or disharmony.

Soon after embarking on this awakening journey, I attended a course about interpersonal relationships – nicknamed aptly, 'A Kick in the Pants'. This workshop was intensive and very revealing. Dad died when I was six years old, and my mum passed when I was in my forties, and this workshop definitely provided support and tools to work through the conversations I so wanted to share with my parents. I always questioned: why had dad left me so young, why did his twin sister survive and remain unmarried, and why could I not have my dad here so that my sister and I could be daddy's adored little girls? It became apparent with the workshop activities there was an opportunity to express these questions and so much more. The power of some exercises was at the core of all my everyday relationships. This confronting workshop equipped me with tools and support to transform my interpersonal relationships on many levels. I recommend that if you want to resolve parent/sibling/partner concerns, this course will assist. I cannot share all of what occurs, as that takes away the surprise and the opportunity for learning. What I can share is that even though my parents had died, and there was no opportunity for a face to face conversation, I could express all my feelings onto paper. Not only during the course, but also afterwards, it became an action where I wrote many individual letters to my mother and father. I would rip them up and start again as I further distilled the content. I embraced this part of the process as it allowed me time to process relevant events in my life that I wanted to share with them and I wrote my absolute honest feelings – the hurt, the sadness, the loneliness and the missed opportunities. Thus, it allowed me to find my voice through the written word. My voice was also heard through the microphone technique. I would hold my pen like a microphone and speak into it as if my mother was in front of me. The combination of these tools allowed all the deep emotions to bubble up and be released. It was a time of being truthful. In my vulnerability was my strength.

Several months after this course, I awoke one morning to realise that my mum had rejected me – belatedly understanding that in my fiftieth year was shattering. I called my boss to advise that I would not be at work that day. Through the tears, I was able to tell him this confronting situation that impacted me significantly. It felt as though I could finally understand why my sister didn't have quite as hard a time at home as I had endured. I must have been in denial or very slow not to realise the situation. Nonetheless, it was about me. Grief showed up as tears flowed as I tried to come to grips with this massive realisation. My mother had rejected me in the final weeks of her death: this was devastating. I became acutely aware of the memory of her anger through the tense facial expressions. If her physical body had any strength, then I would have felt the full wrath of that anger. She tried, yet her arms did not have mobility. It was a time where I plunged into sobs and more questions – *why?* I felt further scrambled, yet the new comprehension somehow gave me clarity. I wasn't only rejected on her deathbed – I had been rejected all my life. Slowly, it was sinking in.

When I look back to my teenage years, I think I must have concerned my mother no end. I probably exhibited a slight rebellious streak within me. More than likely, we all do as teenagers, and I was just average. I had a steady boyfriend, Andrew, and my mother would shine the torchlight onto us as we sat in the front seat of his car, chatting and kissing. Gosh, was it humiliating. My mother never had proper verbal discussions with me; instead, she would write long letters quoting passages from the Bible. These would be on my pillow, silent accusers, when I returned from a night out. There were pages of scripture cited, as well as how a 'good girl' should behave. On the rare occasions my mum would have a discussion with me it would quickly descend into an inquisition. I recall one horrific incident when my mum was questioning me in our kitchen with my sister present. It escalated quickly and my scream pierced the room as my mother's hands seized me around my neck, strangling me with all her strength. It was a shuddering moment fully seared into my memory. On reflection, my mother was distraught after finding that her nineteen year old daughter was taking the Pill. My sister and I were shocked at how a conversation unravelled to a substantial, physically abusive consequence. My sister has since told me she was ready to call the police. This experience was enough for me to consider leaving home, and eventually, I fled overseas to avoid living in this environment. This memory bothered me for many years, and if anyone moved to put their hands near my throat, I would freeze and have flashbacks.

My boyfriend Andrew's mum Dora was so supportive during this period of upheaval. Sadly, not long after, on the eve of our engagement, Andrew had a single-vehicle accident and died. My life plunged into grief. Dora spoke to my mum, asking her to be kind to me as she told us in person of Andrew's passing. I can hardly imagine how a mother who just lost her youngest son could have the courage and clarity to speak to another adult in such a manner. My heart was aching and broken. It took a long time before I could confront what my mother had done to me. Only after my mother's death and doing all the letter-writing was I able to heal my throat. Perhaps mum was mentally unstable to inflict such trauma, yet whatever the reason, physical abuse is not acceptable. Emotionally when a person does not love themselves, it can be very difficult to show love to others.

I moved forward through new-found courage, to go beyond the grief, the pain and reality that had emerged and came to a better place within. Writing letters was an excellent tool to express my feelings and while I couldn't discuss them with my mum face to face, I worked through my emotions writing the letters and reading them out loud as if she was with me. Thankfully, through speaking aloud my written words, I was able to express my feelings, and I came to a peaceful position. Another part of me realised that I chose my parents and all these experiences were part of my life lessons and journey. I always look for the positives and try not to dwell on the negatives as it only lowers my energy, which sends out a low vibration. I want to soar with the eagles and have a high vibration.

I share with you some stories about intimate relationships where it was imperative that I found my voice. Before my full-time university study, I met someone quite special. I wanted to share time together and in time he moved into my home. I was appreciative of his support, both physically with the yard chores as well as the friendship we shared. I became aware that he had stopped his paid work within two months of living with me. Some of the things he told me about himself later proved not correct. I reflected on our conversations throughout his short stay in my home. There was a nagging in my head about the stories; at times, they seemed so far-fetched. Yet I ignored some red flags. He showed me two houses with *For sale* signs and said he owned these and yet there was no way to inspect them, as the homes were rented. Another time he pointed out a boat moored in the harbour – confirming that it was his. While I never confronted him, I realised as time passed that these were his mind follies. In wanting to know his family, we arranged for his daughter to visit. That night the conversation unravelled quite spectacularly over dinner. His daughter's recollection of learning to drive involved lessons with a paid instructor, with no resulting licence as she required more practice and yet in his conversation to me a week earlier he had told me that he gave her lessons and she passed her licence. With such opposite versions of the story, I wondered if I genuinely knew this man. Doubts about my memory from previous conversations with him played in my head.

I spoke up and asked him about the conflicting version of events on his return from dropping her home. He told me 'My daughter was confused' and claimed she didn't remember properly. I reiterated the events. He still maintained his version of events. I felt that his daughter had told the situation truthfully. The next day I listened to my inner voice, my intuition, or as some may call it, a gut feeling. On this occasion, it was not just a feeling, but a loud male voice which spoke powerfully to me; 'Get him out, NOW.' Was I discombobulated? Was God speaking to me? I heard it as a clear strong male voice. I was almost disbelieving of what I heard yet somewhere deep inside, I knew that I had to remove him from my home and life.

Within 48 hours, I heeded these words and prepared a safe time to tell him to leave. It went as smoothly as possible in the situation, although the person did not eat for 24 hours and walked the streets for some time. It was a challenging period, yet I knew it was in my best interests to follow through after such a strong warning. As time unfolded, I learned that this man was not from Zimbabwe in South Africa, as he had claimed – while he had indeed lived there with his parents, he was actually Australian and born in Tasmania. No wonder my inner voice spoke so loudly: there were a considerable number of false stories from this man and for my part, I was so gullible. On reflection, I can see how the stories built a picture of the man he wanted to be, yet sadly his insecurity and these behaviours shielded him from reality and taking action to start anew. No doubt, when so many stories become stated as 'facts', where does one begin to come clean?

Looking at what I could do better, I learned that it is healthier to question things in the moment rather than to let the discussion go unchallenged. Questioning does not need to be an interrogation. It can be wanting clarity and using active listening where you may say; 'I will repeat what I've heard so that I'm clarifying what you just said,' and go into a précis of the subject. Alternatively, you could use the words: 'Let me repeat it back to see that I understood correctly,' or 'My impression of what you said was... is that what you meant?' or, 'So what you are saying is... does that sound right?' Verifying our communication allows us to speak up precisely at the moment, and for those of us who are shy, it takes some perseverance, yet it frees us in that moment. By that, I mean we freely honour the emotion that arises, rather than suppressing the feelings. We speak our truth in the moment. Effectively, we 'nip it in the bud'. What I have learned is that speaking up frees you, empowers you and it clarifies the discussion with the other person. Effective communication incorporates all these tools.

Building that gut communication within oneself is essential. Listening is so critical. I have found that spending time in nature assists awareness of the inner voice, as well as supporting our mental and physical health. We all have chi energy around our being. Let me share a simple 'yes or no' exercise for building and understanding the chi. If you try standing with your legs about shoulder-width apart and knees slightly bent, ask yourself a simple question that requires a yes or no response. For example, 'Is my name X-Y-Z?' The natural chi of your body will take you slightly forward if it is a 'Yes' response and a 'No' response will sway you slightly back. Try it on simple questions first and progressively move to substantive issues. I tried this with a group of underground miners – real salt of the earth type people. I was delivering a session on a very dry Human Resources policy of understanding discrimination, victimisation, workplace bullying, and associated legislation. I asked all twenty-eight attendees to stand and try it. Several of them said that works – of course, it works.

For a long time, I worked predominantly in the Resources industry: corporate offices, operational sites and project environments. In the project environment, our HR department provided courses to bring teams together to foster positive groups who would improve production targets, with dedicated day training on topics like Assertiveness and Communication, Customer Service and Time Management. The feedback from course attendees identified better communications within the team and a new confidence moving forward in the fluid project environment. It was essential to focus on the team, to successfully weave these divergent groups together from different backgrounds and acknowledge the range of cultural customs and corporate values. Everyone who worked on the project commented at their exit interview that they would miss the people – we enjoyed an incredible team spirit which built a high work culture. When exiting an organisation, the exit interview provides a chance to voice your observations about the positives and negatives of the work environment. Completing the exit questionnaire allows input towards potential improvements, plus reinforces what's done well. Speaking up helps self-reflection as well as an opportunity for the business to hear your experiences.

My life often felt like being on a treadmill – continually walking or running from one event to the next with little time for myself, as work was my life. I enjoyed a challenge, and the project indeed extended my skills on many levels, hence giving me limited time for inner reflection. Projects have a start and end date and lots of challenges in between. It was a time for business self-growth learning about ROI (return on investment), delivering analysis of information and submitting recommendations for approval in complex situations. I thrived on these challenges, performing together with skilled professionals who provided stimulating dialogue and awareness to cultural differences.

While I was in Canada for the project work, my son was living in London. I suggested that he visit me as my accommodation would allow him to stay. It was a wonderful reunion, and we managed to take a day trip to Niagara Falls. I was astounded by the size of the falls, and the 'Maid of the Mist' boat voyage gave us an experience of the volume of water spray firsthand. Memories like these are priceless. My son and I departed on the same day as we returned to different parts of the world. He lined up to deposit his luggage and get his London flight seat allocation, and I suggested that I do the same for my Australian flight and then said I'd see him soon. I walked quite a distance and found the correct area, and I kept looking back to see if he was in my queue. I became anxious as I didn't see him. I kept progressing forward. I kept looking back, and at one stage, security pulled me over to check my suitcase.

After formalities, I was seated in the waiting area and asked the staff was there another section, as I wanted to see my son. They kindly explained that in fact, we were in different locations of the airport terminal and that we couldn't wait in the same area. I was shattered and tearful. Minutes later, I was paged. My wonderful son had managed to speak with me to say goodbye via the internal communications. Joyful tears appeared. Relief that at least we spoke yet I didn't have the physical contact, and I knew it would be a good many months before I saw him again. Looking back on it much later, I realised that I must have looked 'suspicious' to the security officer's trained eye, yet I was a mother who hadn't hugged her son nor kissed him goodbye. Speaking to him at least was soothing.

From project life to operational site work in Townsville, I was head-hunted for a role in Brisbane. It seemed a good time to relocate and be living closer to my family, who were now all in Brisbane. I also felt like a perfect time to try an online dating site. I was linked to a few men's profiles as a good match and enjoyed coffee and chats, and finally, I met someone whose values and interests were similar.

During our time together, something wasn't working for me. I couldn't articulate just what, yet we had several heated discussions when this man would berate me or question my opinion. One particular instance was at a restaurant when I asked the waiter what type of vegetable was served with a meal. This innocent question prompted him to speak caustic remarks to me about why I would want to know the type of vegetable and how it was not appropriate to question this in a restaurant. After leaving the restaurant, the barrage of words continued and as I voiced my rationale, it did not matter to him. Sometime later, as small instances like this continued, I wrote a letter to say that our relationship was not working for me and it was best that I leave. He read the letter and we discussed the letter's content. This man suggested that I keep the letter and that we should stay together. Being emotionally connected, I was persuaded to give it another go. Amazingly, a strong woman like me could listen to the placating, subtly patronizing words of his reasoning, in terms such as, 'You are tired and over-reacting,' and I felt swayed into staying. It was a whirlwind romance with lots of activity and at times an aspect of being kept small.

I have found in my lifelong journey that the life-lesson is amplified each time I do not understand it or take action. After a brief period of living together, I found myself tearful and emotional and it felt like I was constantly walking on egg-shells. I experienced the purported love of my life switching from kindness and loving words, to insults and sarcasm in an instant. I became terrified of what might set off an outburst from him. It was deeply unsettling. The daily psychological fear was devastating and debilitating. I was perpetually in a state of nervous anxiety. He vetted what I was wearing daily – I became aware that this was controlling behaviour, and nothing to do with how an outfit looked. These moments had me frozen, unable to grasp the conflicting words I heard and doubting my self-worth. I felt that even on the occasions I dared to speak up, there was rarely an acceptable answer.

A good friend pointed out to me that this man often wanted me to consume alcohol with him and my refusal was never an acceptable option and caused friction. Reflecting back, I could see the pattern and it was one that, for me, felt very destructive. That light bulb moment catapulted my resolve to remove myself from the situation as soon as practical. I am thankful that I was able to escape quickly and start the road to recovery. I met with friends on that decision day, and on stepping out of their spa, I slipped on the concrete. It was a life metaphor – I was falling, hitting the ground hard, sustaining various severe, bruising injuries – the message was not lost on me. I took responsibility for my life and made the choice to leave the relationship.

Transformation came with some sessions provided by a healer who took me back to my childhood, where I found my first point of pain. I now know that, from that point of pain, each time a situation occurred in my life where I thought I was not good enough or not worthy, that I would revert to that little girl of three years old who felt that her parents did not love her. During the sessions, I became aware of my mother and father holding my little sister and being very worried about her health, as she had croup. Across the road lived a doctor, and my parents needed to get medical help as the situation was acute. I had come out to the dining area and saw them, and in their concern for my sister, they hadn't even seen me, and I felt that I was not loved. Deep in my psyche lay this feeling of being unworthy of their love, yet during the breakthrough session, I knew that my parents loved me very much.

These very worthwhile sessions had the healing energy that I required to work through the layers of emotional build-up. It was after working through this first point of pain that I became more aware of how I reacted to others and how I could better understand my role in several relationships throughout my life. Acceptance of myself at that time and the present was, and is, instrumental to my healing and progression of my inner work. I could talk more about the failed relationships, yet it is not about those people; they were the catalyst for me to look deeper into myself and examine 'What was my role?' I know that I can only change myself. This is an important part of my journey and I encourage you to look at your role in any situation. What changes could I have made? What is my choice in this moment? Embrace your intuition and start the change with you.

Again, in each moment, we have a choice, and some of the decisions I made were not what my intuition was guiding me to do. If I wanted to say no, I felt that it was not 'correct' to express that sentiment, and instead would say 'Yes', even though my whole being was yelling 'NO!' It's been a long journey for me to honour that gut feeling – that intuition. I know that intuition does not know right and wrong – what it tells us *just is*. Each of us will receive different intuitive responses – yet it will be the course of action for you only, because it is aligned with you and for your wellbeing. I have read many times that we each have the answers within us – and this is so true.

A simple way to build the muscle of listening to that inner voice is to spend time in a natural environment – take a walk – without any electrical device. Fill your senses with the beauty of your surroundings – sounds and smells and visions of spectacular vistas. Regular time in the bush or beach will provide opportunities for the silence to become a friend. Allowing myself the pleasure of just being in nature somehow stills my soul, nurtures my spirit and enriches life's blessings.

Action Aces

▸ Understand active listening.

▸ Practice active listening responsive lines that feel comfortable with your speech.

▸ Use open communication for clarification.

▸ Ensure the sender and the receiver of communication has equal opportunity to respond to reach an understanding.

▸ Stand and ask yourself a question with a simple yes or no response.

▸ Do you notice the natural chi of your aura? How will you build the inner voice muscle?

▸ Learn to observe your emotional feelings and to FEEL the emotions as they are raised.

  • *Often, we are what I declare, 'into our heads' – our mind thinks about things and replays the situation over and over, and we get to thinking and thinking and thinking! To get out of our head and into our heart is a different environment. As a person who has worked in many business environments, the mind automatically programs the processes, and we think logically, analytically and deliver a program of plans and procedures. I found this a most challenging task; to disengage with my brain and actually to feel an emotion. My brain (mind) kept engaging as it tried to stay in the driver's seat!*

▸ Have you ever tried just sitting with an emotion?

▸ Find a quiet spot now and allow yourself time to feel the emotions within you. When I talk about emotions, I am thinking of love, joy, peace and also anger, sadness, grief. Select one that is current for you now, and just feel, rather than think it in your mind.

- *Can you describe how it felt?*

- *How would you express the difference of experiencing feeling rather than thinking?*

- *What did you learn about yourself?*

▶ Feel into your emotions – rather than utilising the mind – and stay with the feelings until something changes.

▶ Find your voice and a confidante to share what has occurred to you.

CHAPTER EIGHT

Feeling Great
– Believe In You

"Now is the time to be you...
Our greatest journey is our internal voyage.
Take time to discover yourself.
Find your essence, the unique you."

Patrick Lindsay

I love the quote above; each of us is unique. Each of us has a gift – call it a talent – a genius zone. At different times we go about our everyday living and often do not appreciate that particular part of us. Do you know what your talent is? What do you do differently? Does your special gift bring joy to you and others?

I have discovered that even in the midst of my greatest challenges, there are opportunities. I seize these opportunities and focus on the positives that I have gained. I am not putting my head in the sand – I take a proactive approach and flip situations. As a coach, I have learned that if I try one path, and it does not work, try another way!

Experience has taught me to communicate gratitude and appreciation for all that I have learned. Equally, I am thankful for the many friendships I have, which give me joy. Close friends have been with me through thick and thin – these people have spent loads of time listening to me, supporting me with their love and kindness – for this, I am genuinely thankful.

I have learned that I am the only one who can make me happy. Yes, others can contribute and embellish my life happiness, yet ultimately, I am responsible for my state of bliss. Some of my choices have given me unhappiness. I nevertheless appreciate these decisions because they have allowed me to have self-examination. I have read and listened to many people discuss the concept that we each have the answers for what we need to do, inside us. I certainly feel that comment resonates. Even though I believe that we do have the answers within us, part of me will seek an opinion from a trusted person in a specific discipline or healing modality. Perhaps this confirms my course of action or assists me to ponder another new path. I find that a close friend will always speak honestly to me, and I find that refreshing. Sometimes their reframing or curious questioning assists formulation of my next course of action. These close friends never say 'You should do this...' Instead, they kindly offer options and let me decide. I like that openness from my friends as they articulate a summary providing the positives and negatives of each option. I am very much a reflective person, and this method suits me perfectly. I can be impulsive though, as I sometimes feel that this is the way for me and off I go! And so it is. Through this introspection, I realise that I am disposing of old fears and releasing emotional beliefs. My soul has freedom.

I have travelled widely in my life, and I feel very blessed to have experienced cultural differences as well as fantastic cuisine in the most breathtaking places. One particular dream was my wish to visit Antarctica. I always imagined flying over Antarctica for a New Year's Eve treat and so when I was approached to join a trip for eleven nights leaving from Ushuaia in Argentina on a Russian Ice Breaker, my reaction was – what an opportunity – go for it!

Preparation and anticipation are always vital to any trip, as that allows for the excitement to build. Friends gave me books on early explorers, and I read with interest the requirements to take for such a trip. Temperatures were mostly zero and thermal underwear

THE ANSWERS ARE WITHIN

was a must, as well as functional hiking boots and waterproof backpacks.

Ushuaia is the southern-most city in the world, nestled between the Beagle Channel and the Martial Mountains and often referred to as Tierra del Fuego. On leaving this port, I embarked on a journey that not only provided the most breathtaking sights of landscape grandeur and a visual feast of wildlife, but also the heart-stopping moments of winds reaching Force 8 gale levels, the seas a-rockin' and a-rollin' the ship around Cape Horn on the onward journey. Waves breaking over the bridge is a sight vividly recalled – my cabin was located directly below the bridge looking out to sea. Luckily on the return trip, the ocean was like glass and the Cape Horn views amazing.

Nothing quite prepared me for our entry into the narrow Lemaire Channel, where the ice-covered mountains met the inky blue of the water, as the serenity and peacefulness of the early light of dawn at Cape Renard provided a rousing welcome to this continent. Awe and gratitude filled me as much as the silence. I was in shock as no trees existed – subconsciously, while I knew to expect this, part of the Aussie girl who loves the bush was missing the trees.

Gentoo penguins call this area home – the stench of the birds' droppings greeted me before seeing these beautiful creatures in their natural habitat. We set foot on land many times, allowing us to walk around and explore station buildings with the penguins waddling very close. At different harbours and islands, Chinstrap penguins, as well as Adélie penguins, delighted us.

On board, varied talks about explorers, animals, and early ship expeditions provided great insight and a new appreciation emerged for the early explorers' vision and determination. On one particular outing, there were five of us in a Zodiac inflatable boat in Paradise Harbour, and we spotted Humpback whales. Looking in the harbour, many whales performed breaches, spy hopping, when the whale vertically pops its head out of the water, and lobtailing, when the whale lifts its fluke (tail fin) and forcefully brings it down, slapping the water and creating a big splash. These playful mammals decided to have some fun. They came close to the Zodiac. The length of my arm close – and while I could smell the fishy breath, see the barnacles, the one solitary steely hair from the protuberances of the head, lower jaw and pectoral flippers, the whale decided to swim under the Zodiac and come up the other side. Yes, peek-a-boo with a giant of the deep! I was thrilled and excited to have such a front-row seat, yet another part of me felt inner panic, because if we were tipped into the ocean, we had five minutes before hypothermia penetrates. I sat firmly on the Zodiac floor to rein in my feelings, scoring an icy-cold bottom as I contained my emotions. A pod of Orca whales passed by, with Crabeater seals and Leopard seals, at Collins Bay. More penguins were spotted at Peterman Island.

Mother and calf Humpback whales were swimming alongside the ship, while birds flew overhead – Snow Petrel and Arctic Tern – allowing for our senses to be awakened with sounds and our vision to be one of surprise after surprise, sampling nature's gifts. I was thrilled and thankful to observe Minke whales, Weddell seals, as well as the Antarctic fur seal, all safe in their environment. Large icebergs of various shapes dotted the ocean. One looked like a sizeable three-storey bell and another like a large boot with penguins sitting on the toes. Cloud formations provided angelic visions and teased my imagination. As a Human Resources professional, I recall often speaking with managers about certain behaviours being 'the tip of the iceberg'[34] – meaning that the problem or difficulty is only a small manifestation of a larger issue below. Typically, only one-tenth of the volume of an iceberg is above water, due to Archimedes' Principle. It was mind- blowing, observing the icy sculptures towering above the ocean and almost impossible to realise the depth and breadth of what was below. Our

---

34 https://en.wikipedia.org/wiki/iceberg

last afternoon on the Antarctica Peninsula was memorable, with mulled wine and nibbles, and dancing on the stern of the ship, with the thumping 'Twisting by the Pool' music by Dire Straits creating a magical atmosphere. Anytime I hear that song now, my mind wanders to the wonderful wellness of feeling and seeing Antarctica – viewing and appreciating a totally different part of the world where remoteness is valued and honoured. Another life-changing experience and a tick for one extraordinary experience completed from my bucket list.

During and after this adventure, I became aware of my attitude towards gratitude. Antarctica was a dream that unfolded only three months before the travel, and while expensive, it was amazing how the funds manifested for such an opportunity. I gave daily thanks during the trip. Nature is such a big part of my life, and this experience was more than my dreams could imagine. I appreciated the cloud formations in the sky, the sunrise and sunsets, a myriad of seascapes and birdlife, and the people on board the ship who shared their immense knowledge.

Conclusions

Today I give thanks for my loving family, for friendships so warm and precious, especially many people who have supported my journey, the joy of seeing the ocean, as well as the roof over my head and the herbs and vegetables I can grow organically. Life is good!

If you have taken a deep dive into each chapter, you will notice the changes within yourself.

Are you feeling vitality? Taking a small step each day to improve your health makes a big difference over one year, plus the benefits accumulate. Just like cleaning our teeth each morning, it becomes part of our routine. What did you add to your routine?

Have you gained courage? Have you implemented some new breathing techniques to still your mind? Have you taken the time to 'feel' the emotion and let it rise until something within you changes? What step did you decide upon that pleased you most?

How would you rate your self-acceptance? Do you feel that you are more aware of accepting others as well as yourself? If you understand that everything has a frequency, as explained by quantum physics – the desk, the chair and the plate – then how would you rate your own frequency? Do you know when it is low and when it is high? Can you appreciate the importance or calibre of the vibration that is you?

How do you eat an elephant? Bite by bite. And that is precisely how you build confidence. Taking a small step each day helps build our confidence. Looking after how we feel on the inside has an external impact on how we look and feel about ourselves on the outside. What have you noticed about your confidence levels?

Finding our voice is so important! We can sing to the world and convey a message, or we can speak up and share our opinions and thoughts, achieved with respect to another person's beliefs. Honouring oneself is vital to free us from emotional baggage because we raise it in that moment. There are times when silence is golden, yet the majority of times, it is easier to speak up. Keep asking questions of the person who has spoken up so that you are sure that you have received the message clearly.

It can be said that the space between transition and transformation is taking repetitive action daily to ensure the small change becomes a habit.

For some, it is writing through a daily journal to acknowledge thanks. For me, I say it out loud. My strong faith allows me to speak out loud in my car or a solitarily part of my residence with complete freedom. Giving gratitude is one change I made a long time ago and which continues today. I know gratitude is the quickest way to raise my vibration and I feel great. It is the simple aspects of life that provide me with joy and for which I give thanks – things like dance, walking regularly in nature – not only is this a benefit to my physical health, but it is also a benefit to my mental health. Walking in nature also benefits our sleep. Being active encourages so much wellbeing.

Listening to your intuition will give you clear direction, if you listen and follow it. The more you listen and follow, the better choices you make for yourself. Little things like – have you got your keys – might pop up into your mind. When I get this feeling, it prompts me to check that I have keys in my handbag. No, they are on the table! It has saved me a few times by following my inner voice. Remember, build the muscle and follow the prompts, the niggles, as the little things will soon be the very important choices in your life.

Embody the energy of love and allow yourself to receive the gift of knowing The Answers are Within.

Action Aces

▶ What is your gift or talent, and how does it bring you joy? What do you do, to bring happiness to yourself?

▶ Commence a gratitude journal, writing each day what you appreciate and give thanks.

▶ Take time to reflect and voice your 'thank you' to people. Reward your successes – as you work through the exercises, ensure that you celebrate.

Sophia Flowers

PROFESSIONAL ARTIST AND
INTERNATIONAL ART TUTOR

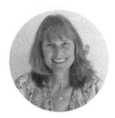

I was aware I was cocooned within a chrysalis and had yet to realise I was a butterfly. It was this realisation that I would set myself free.

My first recollection of art was the paint board my lovely dad bought me – my brother and I would run wildly around the garden and I would constantly go to the painting board and paint whatever I felt. Everything around me was alive and vibrating, full of colour and life.

However, the very same person that gave me the paint board was the one I eventually allowed to squash my joy of creation. At family celebrations, I went to great lengths to create a world of magic, making things and setting a scene. Being on the sensitive side, I still allowed my dad's criticism to affect me. His comments made me feel I wasn't good enough and no matter what I did, I felt I couldn't get it right. Over and over, I felt put down and it hurt. This went on for years, yet initially the joy of painting and creating kept me going until my career choice came into play.

My aim was to attend the local School of Graphic Art and Design, until Dad said that sort of vocation would be hard work for very little money and I'd probably have to live in the heart of London to earn a living. I was a country-loving girl and it was not somewhere

I wished to live at the time. As an adult, I realise this was how my dad was brought up and he too had been stopped from following his dream and because he didn't know better, he was unconsciously doing the same to me. Not knowing any different myself, I took the baton handed to me and believed it. I actually remember standing in the kitchen, listening to him and reaching inside, switching off my light. It was all done very simply and factually because I was by now numb and was having difficulty expressing what I truly felt. Instead it would come out as anger. Even though I believed I had switched off that light, what I didn't know was that it was actually only ever dimmed. It still existed.

Instead of following my passion, the thing that would give me hours of joy and get me bounding out of bed in the morning, I followed a different path, a different vocation and another life. There were relationships, travels, experiences, learning and discoveries about myself... and occasionally the light flickered.

It wasn't until my mid-thirties, when my mum invited me to attend an art holiday with her in Southern France, that things started to change. We arrived in sunshine to a warm welcome from the team and villa owners, where Jo Le-Rose taught us to paint with the Bob Ross wet-on-wet oils technique.

We had a wonderful time with plenty of laughter. The painting though... it was the painting. I loved it. Jo would take us through step- by-step and I would be so absorbed. I felt myself lifting inside and I started to peek over the edge of my self-created box to a view of all that colour. The colour that I so loved, that would sing to me and move, flow and guide me. And so it was, quite simply, standing by the swimming pool in that warm, delightful place that I realized I was home. It was the home inside me and the light was bright again – it called me back to myself. I didn't really know what it all meant; I just knew I was back home within that rainbow of colour. I am eternally grateful to both Jo and Mike Robinson and, of course, my beautiful mum.

Jo Le-Rose, true teacher and gracious person that she is, encouraged me to go and learn to teach this medium for myself. I went to London to do so, loving it all. I was aware I had quite a rebellious nature, having been told what to do so much in my youth, and so I didn't always like to be told what to do at times by those teaching. 'Specific paint worked with such and such medium and best not to do this,' was helpful teaching advice, but why I asked inside. I would return home and practice all that we had been taught over and over, until I had a "Eureka!" moment. Following that, I would let go and do what I had been advised not to and be a bit bonkers. I would splat thinner onto the canvas and allow linseed oil to run and flick the paint at times. I then went on to mix acrylic and inks, introducing them in with the wet-on-wet oil, once dry, coming up with more ideas. It was so much fun and my heart would sing.

Nothing could touch me when painting. It didn't bother me what people thought. In fact, the opposite was happening. Even Dad said some of my art was getting good! My heartfelt love and thanks to him. My artwork was selling within a few weeks and more than one person wanted to buy the pieces. There was no wrong, which was another strange thing when I'd spent the whole of my life trying to be right, be good and be nice, to be liked and loved. I did not care and with that came more freedom. Family, friends and even the postman at the time were buying my paintings – I took it as a sign. I felt humbled and importantly, excited.

And so it was one day that I sat in front of the computer looking at my life. I decided to invest 100% in my art as work and I gave myself a business name, got a simple website up and running and put out an advert to run my first ever painting class. It happened, I loved it and the participants loved it. Since then, I haven't looked back; I'm running Residential Holidays overseas and in the UK, together with painting holiday breaks on the Isle of Wight as well as regular local classes. This has progressed further, to me running classes online to reach a wider audience across the globe. I have done so many things, from murals, to arts and crafts for family holidays, to holding art exhibitions and continually selling work online. It is my wish to continue in allowing that light to move through me to colour this beautiful world of ours and inspire all those with whom I come into contact.

It has been quite a journey. The world didn't suddenly provide me with everything and make me an overnight success. It simply has been one step after the other, and I am the happiest I have ever been, now married and living my dream.

For those that feel they can't paint, I say you can. With someone showing you how and your wish to discover something new, you will surprise yourself. I am always saying the more we don't care about what we are producing, the more incredible the painting becomes. In fact, with my own artwork, the painting paints itself as it emerges from that magical place from within. I love to share that experience with others. And so it was that the butterfly within me slowly emerged from a long, deep sleep and flew off into a rainbow of colour known as home.

If you would like to connect with Sophia, please go to

https://www.sophiaflowers.com/ and

https://www.facebook.com/joyfulpainting/

BIBLIOGRAPHY

Azzopardi, Hollie, *The People Pleaser's Guide to Putting Yourself First*, VIC Australia: Affirm Press 2022

Campbell, Rebecca, *Rise Sister Rise*, Australia: Hay House Australia Pty Ltd, 2016

Chodron, Pema, *When things fall apart*, London UK: HarperCollins, 2005

Coué, Émile, *Self Mastery Through Conscious Autosuggestion*: Original Classic Edition, Gildan Media LLC, 2019

Covey, Stephen R, *The 7 Habits of Highly Effective Families*, NSW Australia: Allen & Unwin 1997

Dryden, Patricia L, *Soul Poems of Love*, Flintshire UK: Protea Printing, 2005

Gibran, Kahlil, *The Prophet*, Oxford England: Oneworld Publications, 1998

Hay, Louise L, *The Power is Within You*, NSW, Australia: Specialist Publications, 1991

Katie, Byron with Stephen Mitchell, *Loving What Is*, New York, US: Harmony Books, 2003

Le Rose, Jo, *Discover Your Full Potential – Live the 7 Steps of How*, UK: Createspace, 2017

Lindsay, Patrick, *Now Is the Time*, Victoria, Australia: Hardie Grant Books, 2009

Lindsay, Patrick, *Be Happy*, Australia: Hardie Grant Books, 2010

Luciano, Yvette, *Soulpreneurs*, Australia: Hay House Australia Pty Ltd, 2018

Martin, Angela, *The Power of Intuition, Trust Your Inner Wisdom,* VIC, Australia: Hinkler Pty Ltd 2021

Nelson, Karen, *How to make money with little money*, Australia, 2020 https://www.smashwords.com/books/view/1010718

Noontil, Annette, *The Body is the Barometer of the Soul So Be your Own Doctor!!*, Australia: 12th Printing 2004

Ricard, Matthieu, *The Art of Meditation*, London: Atlantic Books, 2011

Robinson, Mike, *The True Dynamics of Relationships*, Suffolk UK: Leiston Press, 2002

Robinson, Mike, *The True Dynamics of Life*, Norfolk UK: SOL Promotions, 2010

Schlitz, Marilyn Mandala and Vieten, Cassandra and Amorok, Tina, *Living DEEPLY The Art & Science of Transformation in Everyday Life*, United States of America: New Harbinger Publications and Noetic Books, 2007

Stewart, Margaret, *When THE BIRDS Stop Singing*: Margaret Stewart, USA: 2015

ACKNOWLEDGEMENTS

With the unconditional love of my sons, Leon and Nic, whose love and presence in my life has been significant. Each in their own way and talents, has supported me, and I am so proud of my two beautiful men. Remembering with tenderness and love, the miscarriage of my daughter. Daughter-in-laws, Sandrine and Emily, my love for the beautiful women in our family and wonderful mothers to Lucie and Ava, and Marley, Emily's son.

Honouring Keith Annandale, who is 98 years of age and his late wife, Elsie, my godparents. Words cannot do justice to the support and love they have shown to me all my life. Keith is well respected and loved by many for the beautiful, caring man he is. My life was enriched through their love of the arts and music, to which they introduced me at a young age. Their presence balanced my home life and provided special outings, treats and kindness. My godfather is an amazing man and I am so blessed he is prominent in my life.

To my sister, Leith, mentioned in the book; we share a close bond. She has seen me through all the ups and downs of life and has always given me a listening ear, encouragement and support. I love her dearly.

To my dearest friends, Pamela Taylor and Lorraine Milne, whose love, caring and support has been immense over thirty years. Much love always.

To Mike Robinson and Jo Le Rose, my spiritual teachers whose work is referenced in the book. I have grown as a person by implementing the many tools they have shared in their workshops and online webinars. Their teachings are inspiring and insightful, heartfelt and practical. Much love.

Patricia Dryden, my beautiful soul sister – our friendship bonded instantly in 2010 at the Maldives. Patricia was the first person to read my manuscript and her feedback was so encouraging. Her energetic understanding of words and flow meant the world to me. Thank you, beloved Patricia.

Julia Fellows, a very dear friend and business mentor, who has given me sound professional advice over the years.

To Katrina Duck and Karen Cougan, my dearest Wise Sistar's whose support is appreciated on so many levels. Our bond is strong! Love you lots.

To Karen Tibbits, Tonia Williams and Barb Sinnamon – beautiful friends who have shared my journey very regularly plus the many friends whose love and support has been immense.

To Debi Kearney, Kim Ryan and Lisa Stokx – deep appreciation for holding the light that I would complete this book. With love.

To Sebastian Pagano, for your unconditional love and support over many years. You are appreciated more than words can say. With gratitude and love.

To Pam Day, for giving her beautiful feather photograph to be included in my book. The feather is symbolic to me, and this photo captures the pureness and enchantment so well. Thank you, lovely Pam, for your love of nature and ability to capture it perfectly. Love and best wishes always.

To Karen Crombie, Exact Editing, my editor – recommended by Karen Nelson – you have been a delight to work with and I so appreciate your points of discussion and keen eye. I acknowledge your superb efforts and thank you deeply.

To Sophia Flowers, dearest friend and fabulous artist whose artwork 'Magnificence' graced the front cover of the book's first edition. The joy of colours enriched Sophia's natural calling to paint and her story is briefly told in this book as she truly found the answers within. Thank you, Sophia, for the many pieces of your artwork in my unit – each piece is unique and meaningful, as you are to me.

To Julie Postance, Publishing Consultant and Sophie White, Graphic Designer, my warm and sincere thanks for guiding me on this publication. Each of you have immense experience and skillsets that contributed to this book, and I am very appreciative.

To the many friends whose love and support has been immeasurable – too many to individually mention – know that in my heart you too hold a special place for valued friendship.

Finally, to you, my dear reader, thank you for sharing this journey with me. May you always seek to believe in yourself and know The Answers are Within.

Love,

Anne x